Sarah Ockwell-Smith is the mother of four children. She has a BSc in Psychology and worked for several years in Pharmaceutical Research and Development. Following the birth of her first child, Sarah re-trained as an Antenatal Teacher and Birth and Postnatal Doula. She has also undertaken training in Hypnotherapy and Psychotherapy and is a member of the British Sleep Society. Sarah specialises in gentle parenting methods and is co-founder of the GentleParenting website www.gentleparenting.co.uk. She also blogs at www.sarahockwell-smith.com. Sarah is the author of eight other parenting books: *BabyCalm*, *ToddlerCalm*, *The Gentle Sleep Book*, *The Gentle Parenting Book*, *Why Your Baby's Sleep Matters*, *The Gentle Discipline Book*, *The Gentle Potty Training Book* and *The Gentle Eating Book*. She frequently writes for magazines and newspapers, and is often called upon as a parenting expert for national television and radio.

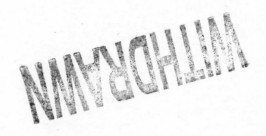

THE SECOND BABY BOOK

SARAH OCKWELL-SMITH

How to cope with pregnancy number
two and create a happy home for your
firstborn and new arrival

piatkus

PIATKUS

First published in Great Britain in 2019 by Piatkus

1 3 5 7 9 10 8 6 4 2

A CIP catalogue record for this book
is available from the British Library.

ISBN 978-0-349-42004-2

Typeset in Stone Serif by M Rules
Printed and bound in Great Britain by
Clays Ltd, Elcograf S.p.A

Papers used by Piatkus are from well-managed forests
and other responsible sources.

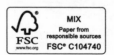

MIX
Paper from
responsible sources
FSC® C104740

Piatkus
An imprint of
Little, Brown Book Group
Carmelite House
50 Victoria Embankment
London EC4Y 0DZ

An Hachette UK Company
www.hachette.co.uk

www.improvementzone.co.uk

For Flynn, my second baby

Author's note

The names of all individuals mentioned in this book have been changed or disguised to protect their privacy.

Contents

Introduction

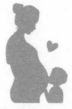

'We're having another baby,' I told my friend after my twelve-week scan. And instead of the 'congratulations' I had been expecting – because that's what everybody said when I announced my first pregnancy – she replied with just three words: 'Wow, double trouble!' This was the moment I realised that having a second baby is an entirely different experience to having a first. Not only do others treat you differently but you feel different, both physically and emotionally, even though you've been there before.

I went into my second pregnancy thinking that I was an old hand – confident and experienced. Just a few weeks in, I understood that while I had been pregnant, given birth and raised a baby before, this was going to be a whole new experience. Yes, I was more confident in some respects: I certainly wasn't worrying about changing nappies, bathing, holding or dressing a baby, as I had with my first. But the space made by the absence of these anxieties was quickly filled with fresh worries: what if I didn't love the new baby as much as my first? Was it even possible to love another child as much? What impact would the new baby have upon my firstborn? I hoped that I was giving him a playmate, a friend for life, but what if they didn't get along? What if I upset his little world? What if he would have been happier as an only child?

And what about me? How would I cope with the pregnancy – the morning sickness and the exhaustion alone – with a toddler to entertain? And the birth: would it be as traumatic as the first time? What would I do with my firstborn when I was in labour? How would I cope in the early days with two children, especially once my partner was back at work? How would I help my two babies to bond? How would I bond with the new baby without the luxury of one-to-one time and without my firstborn feeling left out? How would I ever get out of the house with a newborn and a toddler?

The more I thought about having another baby, the more questions and concerns there seemed to be; and I was supposed to be a seasoned pro! In some ways, I felt more of an amateur than I had with my first. There is an assumption that if you've done it before, you must know what you're doing, so the support for second-time pregnancies is thin on the ground. I had fewer midwife appointments and less contact with the health visitor; most pregnancy, birth and baby books and magazines were aimed at first-timers, as were antenatal and new-mum classes. I had all these questions, but fewer opportunities to ask them. I began to wonder if it was normal to have so many worries second time around. Maybe others coped better than me and that was why the support wasn't there.

Don't get me wrong. It wasn't all negative. Alongside my (many) worries, I had a Waltons-esque picture of life with two children in my head and it made me excited for the future; excited to find out if we were having a boy or a girl and to see what the new baby looked like. Would they have the same big brown eyes and dark brown ringlets as our son? Would they be quiet and sensitive like our firstborn, or more extroverted? What would we call the new baby? I was excited for our little family to grow. Four felt like a nice, even number. I was curious too as to what dynamic the new child would bring to the family. Would I feel 'complete' once this baby arrived? I was so looking forward to newborn squish hugs again and watching the new sibling relationship develop: I imagined two children laughing and giggling in the garden together, and rushing in to wake us up early on Christmas morning; I pictured them in their early twenties, going to the pub together, the best of friends; then, in their late thirties, returning home to us for Sunday lunch with their own families.

So I think it's fair to say my second pregnancy was a strange mix of anxiety, fear, doubt, anticipation, happiness and hope. And I suspect you are experiencing a similarly confusing blend of emotions. But please know that whether you are still at the stage of thinking about having a second baby, already pregnant with your second child or holding them in your arms, those feelings are normal.

My goal is to help you to feel more positive and prepared for life with two children, to gently nudge you towards feelings of excitement, rather than worry. I have tried to include all the questions and issues I experienced myself, and while they might not all ring true for you, you should find that your most pressing concerns are addressed.

Chapters 1 to 3 explore the decision to add another member to the family and when it's 'the right time', what it feels like when that big, fat 'positive' appears (or indeed, takes longer than expected to appear or appears unexpectedly), and the concerns of coping with pregnancy when there's another child to care for. Chapters 4 to 8 cover the practicalities of and planning for labour and birth second time around, especially if your first birth wasn't a positive experience. They also look at how to prepare your firstborn for what's to come, both practically and emotionally, as well as focusing on the period immediately post-birth – the fourth trimester – including establishing feeding and your postnatal recovery, and how all of that looks with two children. The newborn period is tackled, both when it goes to plan and when unexpected circumstances arise.

Chapters 9, 10 and 11 look at the practicalities of life with two young children (otherwise known as 'actually managing to get anything done') and navigating new sibling dynamics. I will propose ways in which you can help your firstborn to adjust to life as a new big brother or sister, how to minimise any difficult behaviour that they may display (as well as how to keep your cool when they misbehave or regress) and how to help your two children grow up with the most positive and close sibling bond possible. Finally, Chapter 12 explores the topic of your feelings as a parent to two – particularly guilt, which will come up time and again throughout the book. I hope to reassure you that almost anything you feel now and over the coming months is totally normal and, more importantly, transient. It also covers the topics of (gulp!) not feeling done at two and gender disappointment.

By addressing these common concerns and questions, I hope to leave you feeling prepared (emotionally and practically), reassured, confident and excited about life with two children. Because, although life as a parent to two can be (and often is) hard, it is also incredibly rewarding and joyous.

A note on using this book

This book is written in chronological order, from making the decision to try to conceive a second baby in Chapter 1, through to discussions about life much further down the line with two children, in Chapters 11 and 12. If you are reading this while baby number two is still a figment of your imagination, then please start at Chapter 1 and read on. I would suggest, however, reading only up to (and including) Chapter 9, for the time being, saving the rest of the book for when you're already a parent of two, at which point they will make the most sense and, I believe, you will get the most out of them. If you are reading with a specific concern in mind, and don't want to read the whole book, each chapter is free-standing; you can dip in and out and read only the chapter, or chapters that are of interest, or concern you, right now.

Chapter 1

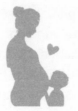

Deciding to Have Another Baby

One of the most common questions I am asked by parents is 'What do you think is the best age gap between siblings?' There is plenty of research looking into the impact of age gaps on family dynamics and relationships. For every study advocating small age gaps, you'll find one warning against them; and for each one claiming that large age gaps are the way to go, you'll find another suggesting that bigger is not always better. There are even studies which tell us the 'best' gap based on the health of the mother. In short, you can always find a study to back up any point of view. But what none of them tells us is what is right for each individual family and their unique situation. Some families thrive with smaller age gaps; others prefer much larger ones. Some don't get to make a choice, finding themselves unexpectedly pregnant with number two. Others need to wait much longer than they had planned or hoped, sometimes giving nature a helping hand.

From my experience of working with families for almost two decades, I have seen that whatever age gap you have, you will cope; you will make the best of it for every family member and, retrospectively, you probably wouldn't change a thing, no matter how you feel at the moment. Different age gaps bring different benefits and challenges. My aim with this chapter (and indeed the rest of the book) is to help you to understand what the science theory says, but, more importantly, how different age gaps may work for you.

The best time to have another baby: what the science says

The more I research parenting, the more I feel that science is unpredictable and somewhat unreliable in terms of studying behaviour, relationships and feelings. The research into sibling spacing is no different, so as I take you on a quick whistle-stop tour of the evidence around sibling spacing, I'd like you to keep this in mind. Consider the evidence when deciding about conceiving baby number two, but more importantly – listen to your heart too. And if you're reading this having already conceived your second baby, please don't get too bogged down by this research, question your decision or worry about the hand that fate has dealt you. Remember, the researchers don't know you or your family. Having never met you, they cannot really tell you what's best for you and your children.

The best age gap for the firstborn

For many years, scientists have been debating the best age gaps between siblings, the focus almost always being on educational attainment and intelligence. The most famous of these theories comes from social psychologists Zajonc and Markus, who conducted a birth-order study in 1975 of almost 20,000 teenagers. In their paper, they argued for larger age gaps between siblings, stating that negative effects of birth order on intelligence and educational attainment 'are mediated entirely by the age spacing between siblings'.[1] They argued that the closer the age gap, the less time the firstborn spent intellectually engaged with their parents.

Findings from a longitudinal study conducted in Hawaii, looking at almost 700 children and following them into adult life, found that an age gap of less than two years can have a negative psychological effect on the firstborn child, particularly in terms of resilience.[2] Researchers believe this is due to them having less time as the full focus of their parents. In contrast, a survey of 1700 teenagers found that an age gap of either less than one year or more than five was the best psychologically for the firstborn.[3] Very small or much larger age gaps, it said, helped the firstborn to feel more positive about themselves and hold less resentment towards their sibling.

Drawing conclusions based on such conflicting research is tricky. The only thing that scientists tend to agree on is that an age gap of around four years is usually the most positive for the firstborn child. This is interesting when we think about natural spacing, or rather what would happen naturally in a world without contraception or formula milk, in which natural-term breastfeeding (breastfeeding into late toddlerhood and beyond) is the norm. While modern-day society makes it tricky to research this in humans, research into the birth spacing in other primates (specifically orangutans, chimpanzees and gorillas) indicates average gaps between offspring of between three and six years.[4] Studies of modern-day hunter-gatherer tribes, such as the Gainj of Papua New Guinea, have found an average gap of three and a half years between births.[5] The marriage of nature norms and psychological research findings would seem to favour slightly larger age gaps.

The best age gap for the second-born

Research indicates that the health of the second-born baby is statistically better if the mother waits at least eighteen months from the birth of her first before conceiving again.[6] Scientists have found an increased risk of neonatal and infant death if the space between pregnancies is less than two years.[7] Nobody really understands why a shorter age gap can have such a negative impact on the health of the second-born, though many speculate it is due to the mother's nutritional status and a potential deficiency in macronutrients or trace vitamins and minerals – these having been depleted during her first pregnancy and postnatal period and not yet having had the chance to fully replenish. While these findings can be shocking, you should understand that we are talking only in increased risks, not guarantees. Every day, thousands of women give birth to perfectly healthy babies who have a small age gap between them and their older sibling. We also need to contrast these findings with those that suggest that larger pregnancy spacings can present their own problems. Indeed, the same research that found problems with a gap of less than two years, also found a higher incidence of premature birth and low birth weight if there was more than four and a half years between conception and the last birth.[8] Purely in terms of physical health, therefore, science seems to suggest that the best outcomes for the second baby occur when there is a gap of eighteen months to four years between pregnancies.

And what about psychological health? The same research discussed on page 9 for firstborns also applies here – favouring larger, rather than smaller gaps for the best outcomes for the second child.

The best age gap for the mother

If a mother conceives again before her firstborn is eighteen months old, research suggests that she will face a higher incidence of premature rupture of membranes (waters breaking), placenta issues (such as abruption, where the placenta prematurely detaches from the uterus, and placenta praevia, where the placenta grows over, or very close to the cervix, the opening of the uterus), an increased chance of uterine rupture if her first birth was by caesarean and an increased risk of pre-eclampsia.[9] Alarmingly, research has found that mortality risk later in life (between the ages of forty and seventy-three) is higher for both mothers and fathers when the gap between their children is less than eighteen months.[10] These parents also require more prescription medication than their counterparts who have children with larger age gaps. Those with *much* larger age gaps (over four years), however, also have a higher mortality risk.

The science here appears to agree with research looking at the best age gaps for the children themselves; i.e. that somewhere between an eighteen-month and a five-year gap is ideal. Science is only one part of the picture, though, and as I mentioned at the start of this section, the researchers don't know you or your personal circumstances. So while research can help us to make an informed choice, particularly with respect to the outcome for our physical health of different age gaps, it can never provide us with a definitive answer. This decision is one that must be as individual as your own circumstances are.

So far, we have focused mostly on the potential risks of certain age gaps. Now let's look at the benefits of different age gaps and the experiences of real-life families who have 'lived' them, including my own.

The top ten benefits of smaller age gaps

'You've got your hands full.' This is something that every parent of children with small age gaps will get used to hearing. My favourite comeback to this is: 'And my heart too.'

Small age gaps are not for everyone. They can be exhausting and require military-style planning, but they can be incredibly rewarding and provide several benefits:

1. **Getting the sleepless nights out of the way all at once** Close age gaps mean that your body is used to frequent night waking. The likelihood is that either your firstborn will have only just started to sleep through the night when baby number two arrives, or perhaps they will still be waking regularly. It may sound like a strange benefit, stringing all the sleepless nights together, but once you're used to the lack of sleep, it doesn't seem like too much of an issue to add another year or two, knowing that you won't need to go back to this stage again in the future. Similarly, the exhaustion of nappy changing, potty training, weaning, teething and developmental spurts and leaps are all over and done with in a relatively short time period, rather than being stretched out over many years.

2. **Reclaiming your home more quickly** When your children all go through the baby and toddler phase at a similar time, your home will look more like a page from a baby-equipment catalogue than an interiors magazine. True, the plastic toys, bulky high chairs, bouncy seats and blocks that litter your floor will be there for four or five

years, but then you will be able to regain a sense of adult normality again. The dirty handprints on every door-frame, crayon wall decorations and unidentifiable sticky substances on every surface will disappear for good, and the cream carpet that was such a silly choice with toddlers will suddenly become a viable alternative again.

3. **Sharing toys and equipment** When your children are of a similar age, they can share the big stuff: climbing frames, ride-on cars and even games consoles in later years can be used by both children at the same stage. Yes, they will need their own toys but a lot of the big, more costly stuff can be shared, reducing expenditure.

4. **Shared interests between siblings** When your children are a similar age, it's more likely that their interests will align, meaning fewer fights over watching *Peppa Pig* or MTV. Family activities are also easier to plan when the children are all into trains or princesses, superheroes or dinosaurs at the same time.

5. **Less potential for sibling rivalry** If your firstborn is very young when your second baby arrives, the chances are they won't remember being your only child. Potentially, this means the transition may be less difficult for them, with less jealousy, difficult behaviour or sibling rivalry in the early years.

6. **Siblings growing up close in age** With close age gaps your family all grows together, which means your children will share their early years and their teen years, going through their university or college or early career years together and then, later, possibly starting a family at the same time. By sharing life experiences in this way, they may support each other more and form a closer bond and friendship as they age.

7. **Less career disruption** Having children close together means that your maternity leave will be taken in a more condensed period of time, with perhaps only a few months back at work before your second leave begins. While this could be disruptive in the short term, once you return to work after the birth of your second baby, the uninterrupted time will allow you to focus fully on progressing your career.

8. **Attending the same schools at the same time** Aside from being practically easier if children attend the same school at the same time (meaning only one school run), they can also support each other at school and may even share friendship groups.

9. **Simpler childcare choices** Children of a similar age are more likely to be together in the same room in a nursery or may share a childminder or nanny. Smaller age gaps can also mean not having to juggle school 'wraparound' care, with a different all-day childcare provider for the younger child.

10. **Fertility or age issues** If it took a long time to conceive your first baby, or perhaps you needed fertility treatment, trying to conceive again sooner rather than later makes a lot of sense. Similarly, if you feel that your biological clock is ticking, and that age isn't on your side, a smaller age gap is an obvious benefit.

My story

I'm an only child and I lost my own parents when I was in my early twenties. As the only member of my immediate family alive, I knew that I wanted more than one child, to prevent my child from feeling as alone as I did. So even before my first baby was born, I was certain I wanted to add to our family quickly.

When my son was born, I was pleasantly surprised at how well I coped. I don't know what I expected life as a new mum to be like, but I must have been pretty pessimistic. As it turned out, I was lucky to find breastfeeding quite easy and emotionally I felt very content and calm, despite a traumatic birth experience. I was in my mid-twenties and fit from regular yoga classes. My physical recovery after a natural (albeit unpleasant) birth was quick, and although I was breastfeeding exclusively, my periods returned at twelve weeks postpartum. When my son was six months old, my husband and I decided to try for another baby. I had resigned from my job; having told them I didn't want to return at the end of my maternity leave, and it felt like we had every reason to add to our family quickly and no real reason to wait. Four weeks later I took a positive pregnancy test, having fallen pregnant the very next cycle.

My early pregnancy went well. I felt very little nausea or tiredness and I focused on raising my son. Because of this, the weeks whizzed by. First time around, each trimester felt like an age and it seemed like I had been pregnant for ever. This time, the pregnancy felt much shorter. However, the latter half of the pregnancy was not so easy. My son was an early walker; he started to walk at ten months old, just as I hit the big and uncomfortable phase of pregnancy. Chasing around after an energetic toddler in the later stages of pregnancy is not fun. Then I started to experience pelvic-girdle pain, my son's hyperactivity increasing as my own mobility decreased. Finally, the very end of my pregnancy was tricky as I developed pre-eclampsia and had to be hospitalised. (I know now that small age gaps significantly increase the risk of pre-eclampsia.) We muddled through though, with a lot of help.

When my second baby was born – another boy – my firstborn was one day short of sixteen months. We'd had discussions and read books together, but I don't think he really understood the concept of another baby arriving. And although I was worried about this beforehand, I think his lack of understanding really helped. He accepted his brother immediately and there were no jealousy, behaviour regressions, tantrums or tears over the new baby – perhaps because he didn't really remember life beforehand. This continued through my second-born's babyhood and we didn't notice any sibling rivalry for at least two years. Our second-born slotted into the family with ease, we already had all the equipment that we needed and growing up close in age meant that the boys had common interests and activities. They shared a room and napped at the same time, giving me some much-needed child-free time. I found it such a positive experience, that when my second baby was five months old I was pregnant again with number three (and number four two years after that)!

There have been times when I've questioned the decision to have children with small age gaps, but I think I would have questioned opting for larger gaps too. Raising children close together has been exhausting and hard work, but now we're all coming out of the other side together. For our family small age gaps have worked well. For others, I know it wouldn't, but all we can do is to consider our own personal circumstances and make the choices that feel right for us.

The top ten benefits of larger age gaps

We know that science generally supports a larger age gap, but by no means is that the only reason to consider greater spacing between siblings. Here are some of the top reasons for choosing to wait before welcoming baby number two:

1. **It allows children more individual attention** Perhaps the best benefit of a larger age gap is the opportunity to give each child more of your undivided time and attention. The first three years of life are often considered the most important in terms of parental affection and attention. Waiting until your firstborn is at least three or older means that you can devote yourself fully to their baby- and toddlerhood. By the time your second baby arrives, your firstborn will be at school (unless you plan to home educate), allowing you undivided time to get to know and bond with your new baby. Fulfilling these needs one-to-one in the early years reduces the chance of sibling rivalry, as each child is more likely to feel that they get, or got, what they need from you.

2. **Easier preparation of the firstborn child** Trying to prepare a toddler for the arrival of a new sibling is a tough task. With limited communication skills and understanding, it's impossible for them to grasp the enormity of what's going to happen to them. Older children have more developed levels of abstract and hypothetical thinking, meaning that their understanding is greater and any preparation you do should be more successful – a more prepared child is more likely to respond positively to the transition once the new baby arrives.

3. **A ready-made helper** A larger age gap means that your firstborn will probably be better able – and more willing – to help when the new baby arrives. Don't underestimate the help a young child can provide, from fetching a clean nappy to entertaining the baby while you prepare dinner. Often, their input is invaluable.

4. **Greater potential for career progression** A larger age gap enables longer periods at work without interruption. That means more scope to climb the career ladder in between children, or time to complete training or further education.

5. **Less sibling rivalry as the children grow** As children get older, a larger age gap can allow them to develop their own interests and friendship groups. Differing interests can mean less bickering over activities, and fewer, or no, shared toys give children a sense of ownership that helps them to feel more positive about their sibling.

6. **More time to restore your fitness and weight** There's no denying that pregnancy, birth and breastfeeding take their toll on the body. I've always thought the saying 'nine months on, nine months off' was ridiculously optimistic – because you spend at least the first three to six months of those nine months in a baby bubble. More realistically, we're talking years and not months to restore your body, regain fitness and lose baby weight. Waiting until you are more 'you' before having another baby is a common reason to choose a bigger age gap.

7. **Makes the joy last longer** Small age gaps may get you through the exhaustion and trauma of baby and early childhood more quickly, but they can also rush through the joy. If you're caught up in all things pregnancy, baby and toddler at once, time passes quickly and, before you

know it, your children are all teenagers and the joy of 'little parenting' has been and gone. Larger age gaps give you time to drink everything in and enjoy every sticky moment.

8. **A more relaxing pregnancy and fourth trimester** There's no denying that pregnancy while raising a baby or toddler is not the easiest experience in the world. Waiting until your child is older, a little calmer, sleeping through the night and with better understanding means pregnancy and the immediate postnatal period is usually more enjoyable and less stressful. If your firstborn is old enough to be at nursery or preschool, it also means you'll have time to relax and nap in the daytime when the exhaustion kicks in. Spacing pregnancies further apart can also help them to feel more special, rather than a chore to be endured.

9. **Less maternal guilt** Regardless of how big or small the age gap, you will always feel guilty when your second baby arrives. Waiting a little longer can, however, ease the feeling of not being able to meet your firstborn's needs any longer or depriving them of some of their babyhood.

10. **Time to save** Financial considerations may seem heartless but they are an important part of deciding to have a second baby. Waiting a little longer gives you time to save, allows you to spend on any big jobs or purchases that are needed before the added expenditure of a new baby, or time to build up a nest egg to see you through longer parental leave, or perhaps switching jobs, reducing to part time or not returning to work at all after your second baby is born.

I asked some parents who had larger age gaps about their experiences and what they would share with other parents who were considering – or facing – bigger intervals between children. Here are two of their stories:

Abby's story

We've got a twelve-year age gap between our two boys. Both children were planned; the second just took a lot more time to arrive. We were actively trying from when the first child was three years old, but after four miscarriages and five rounds of IVF, we decided it just wasn't meant to be. Then, a few months later, we found I was pregnant naturally!

Luckily, our first child has always wanted a sibling, although we were concerned during the pregnancy that he didn't really understand what he was asking for. He was very attentive and helpful though, even accompanying me to midwife appointments and listening to the heartbeat. We would talk openly about our feelings and make sure every conversation wasn't about the baby.

Once our second child was born, he was so excited to finally have a brother, doting and wanting to help where possible. The big age gap meant that he had a better grasp of what was going on, and knew that although we had given him all our love and attention on a one-on-one basis before his brother was born, during the early few months the baby would take up a bit more of our time, while he was still loved and valued. Luckily, we've not yet seen any jealousy. The first child is becoming more independent and self-sufficient; he likes playing with his brother, but he also likes going out to play with his friends. I know the boys will not grow up playing together, but they have their own special bond, which I'm sure will continue to grow stronger over the years.

Deciding on an age gap is a personal decision, and what matters most is that everyone is loved and cared for. The big age gap works well for us, as we've been able to include the first child in all aspects of his brother's life, even down to being there for the birth, which we thought would help with bonding. To anyone who is considering a larger age gap, I'd suggest talking to your child openly and including them in the pregnancy. They will feel more involved as a family member, which will help with bonding, both with parents and with the new arrival. It will also help the older child to still be a child as they play with the younger one, which is adorable to watch.

Catherine's story

Before we had our first baby, we thought that we'd have our children close together, to avoid prolonging the years of limited sleep and total dependency. 'Once you're in a muddle you may as well stay in one,' a friend of mine says. When our daughter arrived, I remember us both talking about having another child soon, having found the birth and early days quite euphoric and addictive. However, our expectations that sleep would improve as time went on turned out to be completely unrealistic. Months six to twelve in particular bring up quite painful memories of pure and utter exhaustion, guilt at not enjoying her as much as I felt I should and challenges within my relationship with my husband. I became obsessed with anything that might affect her sleep and resented my husband because I was breastfeeding so frequently in the night I felt I was doing it alone. He, in turn, felt alienated when all I talked about was her sleep and breastfeeding difficulties. When I went back to work part time when she was thirteen months old, I was forced to night wean as she was waking every one and a half hours and I couldn't function. This actually went really well because even though she continued to wake a lot, suddenly my husband was able to do so much more to help, and with a little more sleep under my belt I was able to think (slightly) more rationally about what was happening.

Until this stage, if anyone brought up the subject of a second child, the pair of us would literally shudder. I could not have imagined anything more horrific! But when she started to sleep a bit, we began tentatively to discuss it, although I felt I needed the time to 'enjoy' my daughter that I had missed out on through sleep deprivation. Around this time I had a sure feeling that I was pregnant (unplanned), but lost the baby very early on – a chemical pregnancy. Despite the trepidation at coping with a pregnancy at this point, I felt very sad. My husband was less affected as it was such an early loss, but we both became surer that we were nearly ready for round two. We planned to try again when our daughter turned two and fell pregnant the first month of trying. By then we were both loving toddlerhood with her and the hard times were starting to fade enough around the edges to make us really optimistic about getting a sleeper this time! It all feels so right, and we feel prepared to cope with the worst of times now knowing we've come out the other side once before.

How do you know when you're ready for number two?

I wish I could give you a definitive answer to this question, but I can't. Some people 'just know' that now is the right time; others question their decision right up until their second baby is born and beyond. Some make a very rational decision, weighing up the pros and cons; others focus solely on their heart and instincts.

I don't think there is any one correct answer, and there are certainly no incorrect ones. So what I will give you instead is a breakdown of some of the points to consider when either you don't have that instinctive feeling about the 'right' time or fate doesn't choose it for you. I've divided them into two categories: head and heart. Ideally, these will be in agreement, but often they are not. If this is the case for you, I can't offer advice, because everyone's circumstances are so different but I will say that while I've never met anybody who regretted having a second baby (even though they weren't sure it was the right time, or indeed the right thing to do), I have spoken to those who regret *not* having had one.

'Head' decisions

I asked parents about the practical points they considered when planning their second baby. Here are some of their answers:

Finances

We decided to wait for three years before getting pregnant again. We had a loan we needed to pay off and we knew it would be a struggle with two children. Waiting allowed us to save and clear the loan, which made our second pregnancy and the arrival of our second daughter a much more relaxed experience.

Work

I thought I'd like a two-year age gap, but I started a new job just after my maternity leave ended, so wanted to get up to speed before getting pregnant. In the end we went for a two-and-a-half-year age gap, which has worked really well.

Space at home

Space was really cramped in our old house. So we decided to do a loft conversion before we got pregnant again. I get anxious with lots of clutter and mess and I knew it wouldn't be a good idea to get pregnant while the builders were working. As soon as the conversion was completed we decided to try again and our second baby was born a year later, by which point we had moved into the new loft room and turned our old bedroom into a nursery.

Waiting until the first child is out of nappies

We always wanted a sibling for our daughter, and there were no major changes in our lives that had to wait, so a month or two after she was one we thought we should start trying. It took us five months, which brought the age gap to two and a half years. It was a plus that our eldest was out of nappies before the youngest was born.

Waiting until the first child sleeps better

My second baby is almost eighteen months old now, and there are just over two years between her and my firstborn son. I didn't want less than two years as my firstborn wasn't a great sleeper.

A ticking biological clock

My eldest was two and a half when number two was born. I was told a year beforehand that I had secondary infertility, so it was a now-or-never-let's-just-try sort of thing.

Previous fertility issues

We have a two-years-and-six-weeks age gap. We rushed into trying for number two as number one had taken us four years to conceive, so we expected to have to go through all that again, but then he came along straight away.

Replicating – or avoiding – your own family gaps

My partner and I had a twenty-two-month and a two-and-a-half-year age gap with our own siblings and felt that had worked for us as children, so wanted to replicate it. Before our first was twelve months old it was definitely too early for us to try to conceive again. I feel within a year of birth it's difficult to make big decisions, as your views are influenced by hormones and sleep deprivation. When she was thirteen months old and sleeping through the night, we felt ready to try again. I have read that it takes at least a year to recover from pregnancy and a gap of more than two years has beneficial effects on brain development of the baby.

Weighing up the pros and cons

Some parents, particularly those who like to make rational decisions, find that weighing up the pros and cons of when – and indeed whether – to have a second child and drawing up a 'reasons-to-wait list' a useful exercise.

If you are still undecided, try filling in the blank chart at the back of the book (see page 265), which has space for your notes under the following headings:

- Reasons to wait

- Importance out of 10 (10 being the most important)

- Possible solutions

You might also want to make a copy for your partner to complete, and then discuss your lists.

'Heart' decisions

Some people can't rationally explain their reasons for going ahead with, or waiting to welcome, a second child. They just have a gut feeling that it's the right – or the wrong – time. But some people never experience that gut certainty. Sometimes the stars seem to align, and things just feel right.

I spoke with some parents who told me they 'just knew' it was the right time or decided to leave the decision up to fate. Here's what they told me:

> I have twenty-one months between baby one and baby two. I knew I wanted a second child before number one was even here!

> I became pregnant within the first month with baby number one, so we decided to 'see what happens' with number two. We started trying when my firstborn was ten months old and I fell pregnant within a month again!

> In my head I knew it was the wrong time. I'd just started a new job and my son wasn't sleeping well. Financially things could have been better too. I just had this feeling though, that now was the right time. It was weird, considering everything practically was so wrong! My heart won in the

end and now our baby daughter is here, and I wouldn't change anything for the world.

When our firstborn was a year and a half old I just had this very strong feeling that now was the right time. I can't explain it. I just knew that another little soul was waiting to join us and was getting impatient.

So sometimes your head and your heart agree; other times they clash. If I could give you one piece of advice about trying to decide on the right time, it would be listen to your heart. It's almost always possible to resolve or work around most of the obstacles your head throws at you. In reality there is never a perfect time. There will always be a practical reason to postpone trying to conceive again. Often, there are unconscious fears and doubts that have nothing to do with the reasons we have come up with for delaying conception, the most common of these being previous traumatic experiences during pregnancy, birth and the postnatal period. If you think this may apply to you, see Chapter 6, where I discuss some of the common causes of anxiety and how to prepare yourself for the calmest and most positive outcome second time around.

What if you are unexpectedly pregnant?

So far, this chapter has focused on planned pregnancies and making a conscious and informed decision to conceive baby number two. I'm fully aware, however, that not all readers will be in this position. Surprise pregnancies can be a wonderful and joyous occasion. I know many couples whose second child was an unplanned but very welcome surprise. I have also met many who weren't so thrilled with the news, at least not initially, and I have worked with mothers who were traumatised at finding out they were expecting again – some because it meant they would have to face head-on the demons they encountered first time around and a lot sooner than they had anticipated, others because of a breakdown or difficult patch in a relationship and still others because it felt like the wrong time, whether for financial, practical or health reasons. One thing I can tell you, however, is that each and every family managed to work with the situation that fate had dealt them, every one of those mothers fell head over heels in love with their new addition and none of them would change their second child for the world. For some of them, it took a lot of work to reach this point, but they all got there eventually, just as I know you will too.

I asked some parents how they felt when they found out they were pregnant with a surprise second baby. This is what they told me:

Our second baby was a happy accident. We knew we would have a second child, but wanted to wait until our first was ready for school, so to have a seventeen-month gap was quite a shock.

I found out I was pregnant again when my first was only three months old. I was devastated. I felt like an awful mother. My baby was literally only a baby. How could I meet his needs and those of a new baby? Fast forward two years and I have two very active toddlers who are growing up together. It's hard work, but I wouldn't change anything now.

My first pregnancy was incredibly hard. I had lots of sickness. The birth was very difficult too and after a three-day labour I had an emergency Caesarean. My husband and I decided that we would stick with only one child. We were happy with our daughter and I couldn't face pregnancy and birth again. When I found out I was pregnant again I couldn't stop crying for days. It felt like the worst thing that could have happened in the world. We weren't sure we were going to continue with the pregnancy, but then I had some bleeding at around ten weeks. Seeing our baby on the scan at the hospital changed something in me. I suddenly found myself willing the baby to be OK, when just the day before I had been verging on terminating the pregnancy. Everything turned out to be OK and I gradually came to terms with the pregnancy with the help of my lovely midwife. I was sick again, but I had a lovely, healing VBAC [vaginal birth after a Caesarean], which I think really helped to finally get my head around things. I have such a strong bond with my daughter now, and though it's not what we originally had planned, I can't imagine our lives without her now. I feel blessed that she came along unexpectedly, as without her I wouldn't have had my healing second birth and I never would have been brave enough to try for another baby consciously.

The main thing I took away from the conversations I had with mothers who experienced unplanned second pregnancies was that there is no one right or wrong way to feel. There are myriad complex emotions and every single one of them is justifiable and normal. It's OK to feel negatively towards the pregnancy and even the baby. It's OK to feel excited, scared, angry or, perhaps, jealous of others who haven't had to go through this. Don't feel guilty for feeling, whatever that feeling is.

Practically speaking, I would strongly recommend speaking to other parents who have children with a similar age gap. Ask them how they coped, what they would do differently if they could do things again and what tips they have. If you're not feeling up to doing this in person, then internet discussion forums can be a lifesaver, especially using a pseudonym if you want to stay anonymous.

If you feel you need a little more help, then speak to your midwife or doctor and ask for a referral to a counsellor; or, if money stretches, see one privately. Speaking to a specialist midwife or counsellor can really help you to make sense of your feelings and allow you to come up with a coping strategy and plan going forwards.

Try to keep communication open with your partner too, if you have one. If you find it too difficult talking face to face, then emails, texts or old-fashioned letters can help. Whatever you do, though, speak to *somebody* and share your concerns. You are not the first person to be in this position and help is available. Finally, I hope Becky's story below, about her unplanned second pregnancy, will help you a little.

Becky's story

We planned to leave a gap of two or three years before trying for another baby, and so I had a coil put in at four months postpartum. Just after our daughter turned one, the coil came out unexpectedly – suddenly there it was on the floor of the shower. Because it had taken six months to conceive before, and we reckoned we were much more tired and stressed now, I didn't get another one fitted. We decided we'd just be 'careful' and watch my cycle instead. Clearly nature had other plans because I got pregnant almost straight away. There would be less than two years between our two children.

I didn't realise I was pregnant until I started getting morning sickness at seven weeks. I thought I'd had a period, but I realise now that it was implantation bleeding. One day, I felt tired and nauseous, exactly as if I had a hangover or I'd eaten something bad. I asked my partner if he had the same symptoms, and we went over all the things we'd eaten in the last week. The next day, I felt exactly the same and on the third day I bought a pregnancy test. It came up as a clear, unmistakable positive.

It was much more of a shock than I had expected, both to me and my partner. We didn't really know what to do or how to feel. The first time around we had been overjoyed, yet this time we felt worried, confused, slightly unsure. The baby wasn't supposed to happen this soon. It wasn't the plan. We felt that it was somehow unfair on our daughter to have a sibling so soon, as if she deserved longer with 100 per cent of our attention. We felt that we wouldn't be able to give the new baby the same level of care that we'd given our first. I was worried that my milk would dry up during pregnancy and I would be denying my daughter her morning and evening feeds. Most of all, we felt guilty for having these questions. We felt guilty for not being immediately happy about being pregnant.

It took quite a long time for us to process the news properly. It really didn't help that I was feeling very sick and that at the time we both had heavy workloads. I just wanted to bury my head in the sand and not think about being pregnant. We worried about jobs, and shared parental leave, and whether our childminder had space for another child (and how we'd afford it). We talked about our worries and looked things up online, calculating the cost of future childcare on a spreadsheet. Once the shock had faded away, we realised that we were just as overjoyed at this baby as our first. It wasn't quite what we'd planned, but once we had worked out some of the practicalities we were able to relax and let ourselves be happy about it.

So when is the best time to have another baby? I genuinely believe that there isn't one. Yes, there are pros and cons to different gaps, but ultimately it comes down to what you do, how you prepare both yourself and your firstborn and how you plan for life afterwards. And whatever age gap you end up with, you will make sure it works for you and your family.

Over the coming chapters, I'll help you to do just that. First, though, the next chapter looks at conceiving your second baby. If you are already pregnant, please go straight to Chapter 3, which looks at how to navigate (and even enjoy) your second pregnancy when it isn't – and can never be – your sole focus, as it was the first time around.

Chapter 2

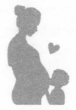

Conceiving the Second Time Around

Having made the momentous decision to try to conceive baby number two, I find that many parents would like more information about fertility second time around. Perhaps their first baby was conceived very quickly, within a month or two of starting to try. Perhaps it was unplanned and a surprise. Perhaps it took several months, or even years, but they conceived naturally. Or perhaps they needed fertility treatment after a long time of trying. Whatever the situation was the first time around, it doesn't always follow that number two will be the same or even similar.

In this chapter I will cover what to expect, no matter how long it took the first time, and what you can do if things are taking longer than you imagined.

How long will it take?

The length of time taken to conceive depends on many factors, including age, health, medical history and lifestyle, combined with a big dose of luck. For every 100 couples (of childbearing age) trying to conceive naturally, 84 will become pregnant within a year. Estimates suggest that around 7 per cent of couples will experience fertility issues.

According to a 2016 study, the chances of conceiving decline with age, as follows:[1]

Maternal age	Chances of conceiving naturally within 12 months
25–30 years	90–95%
30–33 years	83–85%
34–37 years	66–73%
38–39 years	35%
40–44 years	25–33%

With second babies, the simple fact that you are slightly older than you were when you had your first baby can mean that it may take slightly longer to conceive. This is not always the case, though, as we'll find out when we look at some 'real-life' stories later in this chapter. If you feel inclined to start trying earlier than planned, just in case it takes much longer to conceive this time, be aware that it can also happen surprisingly quickly and you may find yourself pregnant sooner than you had planned. Percentages and chances are just that; they are not guarantees!

What if your periods have not restarted?

If your periods have not started again since the birth of your first baby, you may believe that you cannot get pregnant. This is not strictly true. To explain this more clearly, we need to take a quick look at the female menstrual cycle.

The menstrual cycle begins with the secretion of oestrogen and follicle-stimulating hormone (FSH). FSH causes the egg to grow until oestrogen levels rise to a certain point which results in the cessation of FSH secretion. After this, luteinising hormone (LH) is secreted, which causes the egg to be released – better known as ovulation. After ovulation, a period known as the luteal phase begins: following the release of the egg, the empty follicle forms a structure known as the corpus luteum, responsible for secreting the hormone progesterone. In turn, progesterone readies the body for a pregnancy, by preparing the lining of the uterus for implantation and embryo growth. If pregnancy has not occurred, the corpus luteum degenerates and progesterone levels fall after approximately ten days. When they have dropped low enough, menses (or your period) begins.

Ovulation normally occurs around ten to fourteen days before your period starts, as the chart overleaf shows. This means that for your first postpartum cycle, you may well be fertile without realising it – that is, you are likely to ovulate before experiencing your first postpartum period.

Although it is possible to conceive before your first postpartum period, it is common for the first few cycles after having a baby to be anovulatory (without ovulation, or the release of an egg). Postpartum anovulatory cycles occur in an average of 30 per cent of women.[2] Luteal phases are often shorter postpartum and may be too short to sustain a pregnancy, even if conception has occurred. A luteal phase of ten days or shorter can cause lowered fertility because the lower progesterone levels inherent in a short phase are not high enough to maintain a pregnancy.[3]

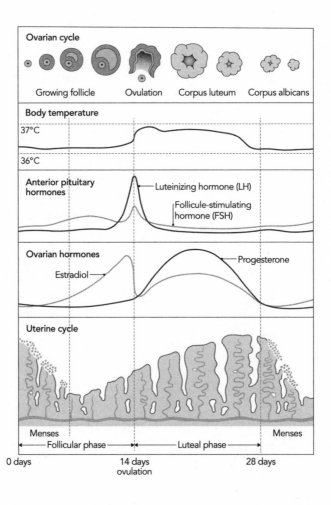

Ovarian cycle

Growing follicle   Ovulation   Corpus luteum   Corpus albicans

Body temperature

37°C

36°C

Anterior pituitary hormones

Luteinizing hormone (LH)

Follicule-stimulating hormone (FSH)

Ovarian hormones

Estradiol

Progesterone

Uterine cycle

Menses   Menses

← Follicular phase →|← Luteal phase →

0 days   14 days   28 days
                      ovulation

What if you're still breastfeeding?

Mothers who are breastfeeding are often advised to stop feeding their firstborns if they want to conceive again. However, this isn't necessary, unless you want to. As I've said, you can still be fertile even if you do not have your periods back, and every year thousands of mothers conceive while regularly breastfeeding. Mothers experiencing lactational amenorrhea (the medical term for an absence of periods due to breastfeeding) still have a 67 per cent chance of ovulating by twelve months postpartum.[4] In terms of when to expect your periods to return – if you are breastfeeding regularly, day and night (or 'on demand' as it's more commonly known), and not supplementing with other milk, then there is around a 22 per cent chance that you will menstruate again by the time your baby is six months, an 80 per cent chance before your baby is twelve months and a 92 per cent chance by their second birthday.[5] If your baby is older than six months, you are not exclusively breastfeeding (i.e. your baby is eating solids), you are feeding infrequently at night and your periods have returned you have a good chance of conceiving, despite breastfeeding.

Although it is certainly possible to conceive while breastfeeding, there is a slightly lowered chance of conception compared to non-breastfeeding mothers. Research has shown that exclusively breastfeeding mothers are more likely to experience an anovulatory period, compared to those non-exclusively breastfeeding, i.e. supplementing with formula or food, or not breastfeeding at all.[6] Exclusively breastfeeding mothers are also more likely to experience a short luteal phase incapable of sustaining a pregnancy than their supplementing or non-breastfeeding counterparts. Full fertility is considered to be restored, and comparable with a non-breastfeeding mother, once breastfeeding is no longer affecting the follicular phase (egg growth), ovulation or the luteal phase. Research has found this tends to happen around the seventh postpartum menstrual cycle.[7]

If you are breastfeeding and would like to speed nature along a little, scientists have found the following may help your fertility to return to normal:[8]

- Keeping the number of daytime feeds to a maximum of three

- Keeping the length of each feed to ten minutes at the most

- Restricting non-nutritive suckling (where the baby suckles at the breast for comfort, but does not really drink milk)

- Restricting or stopping night feeding. There is no recommended number of night feeds, however restricting non-nutritive suckling would apply here. The researchers also found that fertility was most likely to return when total feed time over the course of twenty-four hours was restricted to a maximum of sixty-five minutes. With three night feeds at the most, lasting for ten minutes or less, this would leave two ten-minute daytime feeds and a ten-minute bedtime feed. Some women may find that they need to stop night feeding altogether for fertility to fully return, however.

While these statistics provide a helpful guide, you may find that you can feed more often and for longer and still conceive, or that you need to reduce the numbers given above. (In Chapter 3, we will cover breastfeeding during pregnancy – in particular, how a new pregnancy may affect your breastfeeding relationship with your firstborn and how breastfeeding affects a developing pregnancy.)

Increasing the chances of conception

If you want to boost your chances of conception consider the following steps, which have been shown to help:

- **Lose weight if you are overweight.** According to research, losing weight can improve your chances of conception if you are overweight or obese, with a weight loss of as little as 5–10 per cent of body weight shown to have a significant effect on fertility levels. [9]

- **Eat a healthy diet and take regular exercise.** Research has found that a healthy diet, with a high intake of fruit and vegetables and low intake of fast food, leads to higher fertility rates, compared with one featuring less fruit and vegetables and more fast foods.[10] Exercise matters, too, for both men and women, with regular exercise aiding fertility.[11]

- **Stop smoking.** Men who smoke are known to have a significantly reduced rate of fertility, compared to their non-smoking counterparts.[12] This effect is also seen in women.[13]

- **Get adequate sleep.** Scientists have found that having disordered sleep makes women three times more likely to struggle with infertility.[14] The same statistical link has been found in men.[15] Night shifts and exposure to light at night (from phone screens, for example) can also have a negative impact.

- **Have regular sex at the right time.** It may sound silly, but a common cause of delayed conception is simply not having enough sex at the right time. Understandably with one child to look after, finding time for sex can prove tricky. Tracking your cycle and monitoring your most fertile days can really help, as I will show below.

Fertility-awareness methods

A common cause of a delay in getting pregnant is having sex at the wrong time of the menstrual cycle.[16] Research has shown that up to half of those trying for a baby are unaware of how their cycle works and mistime sex as a result.[17] When looking at the menstrual cycle (see page 35), I explained that ovulation typically occurs somewhere around Day 14. However, this can vary from as early as Day 10 and as late as Day 20 and beyond. When the body is close to ovulating, it produces cervical mucus (which some may refer to as vaginal discharge). This mucus helps sperm to survive. At its most fertile (when it resembles raw egg white), sperm can live for up to five days, but most survive for between one and two days. Shortly after ovulation, the production of cervical mucus ceases and fertilisation chances dramatically reduce. Research conducted in 1995 highlights the six days, in relation to ovulation, when fertilisation is possible, and the chances of conceiving on those days: [18]

Day of intercourse in relation to ovulation	Chances of conceiving
6 days before	0%
5 days before	10%
4 days before	16%
3 days before	14%
2 days before	27%
1 day before	31%
Day of ovulation	33%
1 day after	0%

Tracking ovulation can significantly help to increase the chance of conception.[19] Here are some of the most common ways in which this can be done:

- **Ovulation predictor kits (OPKs)** OPKs look a little like pregnancy tests. They work in the same way, in that you urinate on them. They check for the presence of luteinising hormone (LH) in your urine. LH (see page 36) is responsible for causing a mature egg to be released (ovulation). Testing daily from around Day 10 of your cycle gives you a good idea of approaching ovulation and having sex on days that the OPK shows as positive can help increase your chances of conception.

- **Basal body temperature (BBT) charting** Your body's temperature first thing in the morning, before you move or get out of bed, is at its lowest. Tracking this BBT each morning, with a highly sensitive thermometer or a fitness tracker, can help to pinpoint ovulation retrospectively when you plot results on a graph. On the day immediately after ovulation you have a temporary body-temperature spike of 0.3–0.9°C. So by charting your temperature for a few months, you can usually pinpoint a pattern in terms of the day of ovulation, which can help you to plan on which days to have sex.

- **Cervical mucus monitoring** As mentioned earlier (see page 40), the presence of fertile cervical mucus – thin and stretchy, like raw egg white – indicates the most fertile period of the cycle. Aiming to have sex on days when fertile cervical mucus is present can increase the chances of conception, especially if this method is coupled with BBT charting (see above).

- **Tracking ovulation pain (Mittelschmerz)** Some women feel a distinct, sharp pain or cramp when they ovulate. This can also be followed by a dull ache in the lower tummy, which tends to be one-sided (the side where ovulation occurs). The medical name for this is Mittelschmerz, which is German for 'middle pain'. Mittelschmerz can help identify the day of ovulation, which can allow you to choose which days to have sex on in future cycles. While Mittelschmerz is common and normally nothing to be concerned about, it can also indicate the presence of endometriosis (scarring around the ovaries, where the endometrium – the tissue that normally lines the uterus – grows outside the uterus, often around the ovaries and Fallopian tubes) or polycystic ovary syndrome (PCOS), where fluid filled sacs develop around the surface of the ovaries. These can cause issues with fertility, as I will explain later in this chapter. If you have any symptoms over and above Mittelschmerz it is worth discussing with your doctor.

- **Fertility-awareness apps** Several apps are available which enable you to track your cycles and pinpoint ovulation, usually including BBT and cervical mucus tracking. See the Resources, page 267 for more information.

Finding time for sex when you have a young child

For many parents, one of the biggest obstacles to conceiving a second child is simply finding the time and energy to have sex. Here, my advice is to grab any opportunities. Don't just rely on nights. Night-waking is the ultimate passion killer, and at the end of a long day taking care of a young child, most parents just want to go to sleep. Instead, embrace the silence of daytime naps, and times when your child is at nursery, preschool or school. Or, if you know ovulation is approaching, consider asking grandparents if they can have your child for the day, or weekend (though perhaps don't tell them why).

When conception happens quicker than you expected

From all the mothers I spoke to who found themselves pregnant much sooner than they had expected, or hoped, the overwhelming message was that it's OK to feel whatever you are feeling. Don't feel guilty for not cherishing the new pregnancy or for feeling down that fate has taken control. Allow yourself to feel whatever you are feeling and don't rush yourself to feel otherwise. Nine months is a long time; you don't have to feel joyful and thankful from the start. You may find the experiences of the mothers in Chapter 1, who became pregnant unexpectedly (see page 28), reassuring.

When conception takes longer than you expected

For some of you reading this, it will take longer than you expected to conceive your second baby. Perhaps you already experienced fertility issues with number one and were hoping things would be quicker this time; or perhaps you conceived quickly with your first child and can't understand why things are taking so long now. I spoke to some mothers whose second babies took longer than they had hoped, or imagined, to arrive. Here's what they told me:

It took us four years (and lots of Clomid medication) to conceive our second baby, versus only two months' natural conception with our first.

My firstborn was a happy accident. We weren't trying to conceive. When it came to trying again, I naïvely expected things to happen very quickly. I was wrong. It took us fourteen months to conceive our second baby. We had tests that showed there was nothing wrong with either of us. Nobody could explain why it took so much longer. I guess it was just one of those things.

My daughter was conceived the very first month we decided to try for a baby. We started trying again when she had her first birthday as we were hoping for a small age gap. Never would I have imagined that it would take three years' worth of on-and-off trying for number two to come along. We tried for almost two years and then felt we needed a break from the stress. Nine months later we started to try again, and he was conceived on the third cycle. I was thirty-nine when my firstborn was conceived, so I suspect my age had something to do with how long it took us to conceive second time around. I was forty-three when my son finally arrived.

My first child was born after three miscarriages. I did not need any treatment as all tests came back normal, so somehow, I felt that my body would know what to do when we decided we wanted to have another baby. Unfortunately, I went on to have two further miscarriages, the first after the birth of my eldest being the most traumatic as I felt my body was letting me down – again – but at the same time, I had to keep a happy face for the eldest, who was eighteen months old at the time. After my fifth miscarriage, I decided I was going to give it one more go, as it wasn't fair on my existing child to keep getting depressed and ill whenever a new miscarriage happened. I went to see a specialist doctor and, with progesterone and Clexane medication, I finally got my second child. I couldn't believe it was really going to happen – probably for the first twenty weeks – as I kept thinking something was going to go wrong. This also meant I didn't do any pregnancy announcements and didn't tell my firstborn until I was seven months pregnant when there was no hiding to be done.

Secondary infertility

Research shows that among those who decide to try to conceive a second baby, one in six will not have done so after twelve months of trying.[20] This is known as secondary infertility.

There is a widespread misconception that fertility issues are easier to cope with when you already have a child. Insensitive comments from others don't help, like: 'At least you already have one', or, 'Be grateful you already have a child'. It's OK to want another child and it's OK for feel anxiety, envy and anger if you're struggling to conceive another.

In fact, in some ways, these feelings can affect you even more when you are facing secondary infertility, as you are already immersed in a world of babies. Friends you made at antenatal classes the first time around all start to welcome their second babies; you see babies at nursery and day care, at the park, at soft play. It's impossible to avoid seeing what you're missing on a daily basis, unlike someone struggling with infertility the first time around.

Wanting another child doesn't make you any less grateful for your firstborn (it can even make you more so), it doesn't make you selfish and it definitely isn't easier when you already have a child.

Causes of secondary infertility

Causes of secondary infertility are like those of primary infertility (infertility having not yet had a baby). They include:

- **PCOS** See previous explanation on page 42.

- **Endometriosis** See previous explanation on page 42.

- **Blocked Fallopian tubes** The Fallopian tubes can become blocked due to scarring from surgery, endometriosis or from a previous sexually transmitted infection (STI).

- **Luteal-phase problems** Luteal phases are sometimes too short to sustain a pregnancy.

- **Irregular ovulation** Most female-factor fertility issues relating to the menstrual cycle occur because of problems with ovulating, including not ovulating regularly or even anovulation, where ovulation doesn't occur.

- **Thyroid problems** Both hypothyroidism (an underactive thyroid gland) and hyperthyroidism (an overactive thyroid gland) can impact on fertility, particularly ovulation.

- **Fibroids** These are benign (non-cancerous) growths that occur around and inside the uterus. Their position may block one or both Fallopian tubes or prevent implantation of a fertilised egg.

- **Male-factor infertility** Male infertility is usually down to the quality of semen. Problems may include a low sperm count, poor motility (movement) and abnormal, deformed sperm.

- **Medication** Some medications, such as those used for chemotherapy and non-steroidal anti-inflammatories (for instance, aspirin and ibuprofen), can negatively affect fertility.

- **Advanced maternal age** This is the most common cause of secondary infertility. A woman aged thirty-eight or thirty-nine years old, has roughly half the chance of conceiving each month than she did at thirty-six or thirty-seven (see page 34).

- **Unexplained infertility** This occurs when no other cause is found to account for the difficulty conceiving.

Seeking help

If you are in your late thirties or forties, it is advisable to seek medical help after six months of trying to conceive; if you are younger than this and have not previously had fertility issues, you should get advice once you have been trying for twelve months.

For most, the first point of medical contact for fertility concerns will be your family doctor (GP). Ideally, both partners will attend this appointment. Your GP will spend some time discussing your medical and obstetric history. They will ask you how long you have been trying to conceive, how often you are having sex and about your general lifestyle (including what you eat, how much alcohol you drink, whether you smoke, as well as questions about your job and how much sleep you get). They may weigh you and perform an examination of your pelvic area. Finally, they may order blood tests to check your levels of progesterone (to ascertain if you are ovulating). If these initial blood tests do not indicate any issues, your doctor may decide to send you for an ultrasound scan to see if the problems are caused by something in your fallopian tube, ovaries and uterus, such as a blockage or fibroids. Depending on the results of the scan, you may then be referred to a gynaecologist to help resolve any issues found, or to a fertility specialist if the lack of conception remains unclear.

What treatments are available?

After any diagnosis, treatment will take one, or more, of three routes:

- Surgical (such as performing a small operation to unblock Fallopian tubes or to remove fibroids)

- Pharmaceutical (medication may be given to encourage ovulation or to reduce the effects of PCOS)

- Assisted conception, which can be broken down as follows:

  - Intrauterine insemination (IUI). The simplest assisted-conception technique, IUI involves the insertion of sperm (selected for the best quality) directly into the uterus.
  - In-vitro fertilisation (IVF). The term 'in-vitro' means 'in glass', and with IVF, an egg is fertilised by sperm outside of the body. Embryos that result from the fertilisation procedure are then returned to the mother's uterus.

– Intracytoplasmic sperm injection (ICSI). ICSI is used when sperm quality or quantity is low. It involves injecting an individual sperm cell directly into the egg cell. ICSI is performed alongside IVF.

Funding fertility treatment

If you are in the UK, any tests that you are referred for by your GP will be free of charge on the NHS. If you are not exempt, you will need to pay for any medication prescribed. If you need to utilise assisted-conception techniques, then as a parent already, it is unlikely you will be entitled to NHS-funded treatment. Most local clinical commissioning groups (CCGs) only provide assisted-conception funding for those who do not already have children, although it is always worth checking with your local group to see if the policy is different in your area.

There is no regulation for the fees charged by private fertility clinics, so they are free to set their own prices. Consequently, these can vary wildly (and don't necessarily reflect success rates), but (at the time of going to press) you can expect to pay in the region of:

- £800 to £1500 per cycle for IUI

- £4000 to £8000 per cycle for IVF

- £500 to £1500 per cycle for ICSI (in addition to IVF fees).

Many clinics run payment plans to help to spread the cost of treatment and may also offer discounts for paying up front.

When you select a private clinic, make sure that you visit several of them. Ask to see their success rates for your age group and ensure that they are registered with the Human Fertilisation and Embryology Authority (HFEA) – an organisa- tion run by the UK government, which regulates and ensures standards among UK fertility clinics. There are some useful organisations listed in the Resources, page 267, providing advice and support for fertility treatments.

I hope that this chapter has helped you to understand fertility, and specifically how it relates to second babies. If you are still at the stage of trying to conceive, I recommend that you come back to this book a little further along your journey. If, however, you have recently taken a positive pregnancy test, then please do read on.

Chapter 3

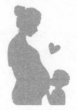

What to Expect When You're Expecting Again

Y ou've been pregnant before, but that doesn't mean that your second pregnancy will be the same. For some, their pregnancies are very similar; for others they are like chalk and cheese. No matter how similar your pregnancies are, however, the one thing you haven't done before is to be pregnant with another child to look after. In this chapter, we'll look at what to expect: your emotions, the physical differences of a second pregnancy, variations in antenatal care, and how to cope with sickness, reduced mobility and exhaustion when you can't sneak off for a nap, as you might have done in your first pregnancy.

When that 'positive' no longer feels quite so positive

Regardless of the circumstances, I think there is always an element of 'Have we done the right thing?' when you are pregnant for the second time. For some, this feeling hits the instant they see two blue lines; for others – like myself – it sneaks up slowly, until one day, perhaps in your first trimester, your second or even third, you wake up with an out-of-the-blue sense of anxiety and think, I'm not so sure this is a good idea.

Whenever this feeling arises, rest assured that it – and you – are totally normal. It's OK to have doubts; it's OK to worry about how you will cope; it's OK to feel a sense of grief at losing the one-to-one relationship you have with your firstborn; and it's OK to feel scared about giving birth again.

I spoke to some mothers about their feelings during their second pregnancies. This is what they told me:

My second pregnancy was a surprise. My son was seven months old when I found out I was pregnant. I worried about how this would impact on his life and I worried about being able to love another baby the same way. I just couldn't imagine it.

I was very excited, but nervous about the labour as my first was traumatic.

I was so nervous when I found out I was pregnant for the second time, as it was unplanned. My little girl was still obsessed with breastfeeding, was still bedsharing with me and at twenty-one months, still not sleeping through the night. This was exacerbated when I found out that I was pregnant with twins! I cried a lot for the first few weeks, as didn't know how I was going to cope with two newborns and, more importantly, how my little girl was going to cope. This changed at my twenty-week scan, when I found out one of my boys had a congenital lung defect and there was a chance that he wouldn't make it. It put it all in perspective. All I wanted then was my three babies together, and I knew we would find a way to cope. I'm an only child and my upbringing helped me to see how lucky my daughter was to be getting two siblings in her life.

It took me some time to come to terms with being pregnant again so quickly. I wanted to totally enjoy our firstborn's first year. I didn't feel mentally prepared for pregnancy again so soon, especially as the morning sickness was so horrid the first time. I had no idea how I was going to cope with a toddler while pregnant. Thankfully, it's not been so bad – so far!

We were lucky to conceive pretty much as soon as we made the decision and were so excited to see those two blue lines. I'd had a straightforward pregnancy and birth the first time around, and had everything crossed it would be the same this time. It never occurred to me that I would feel such strong bouts of guilt. The first time was in the shower, crying my eyes out, thinking of my son and how everything was going to change for him, and he didn't have a clue. He loves it when the three of us are together and he has our sole attention. How is he going to feel when he has to share our attention with another baby? Those feelings came back when the three of us were snuggled in bed in the morning and my son looked up at me with his beautiful, innocent eyes. I felt so guilty that we were about to completely change his whole world, and worried that as little as he is, he might resent us for it. Then I worry about how we are going to cope too. My bump is growing day by day, along with my love for 'Dot'. I feel guilty for loving my unborn bundle. What about my love for my son? He's my world. How can I love both of my children equally? I'm still not sure how to resolve these feelings. They keep coming back to me with floods of tears while at the gym, on the train. The logical part of me knows everything will be fine. One of the reasons we are having another child is because we're sure our son will love having a sibling. I guess it's just all part of the emotional rollercoaster of motherhood.

Coping with your feelings

For most mothers, the worry subsides naturally as pregnancy progresses. Preparation is key here: preparing your firstborn to become a new big brother or sister; preparing your home for the arrival of a second baby; preparing to give birth again; preparing for childcare while you're in labour; and preparing for the early days with two. Preparation allows you to explore your feelings and options in a productive way; it also allows you to feel more excited and calm about your new baby's arrival.

You may need help to prepare and much of the rest of this book is devoted to this. Sometimes all you need is a pen and paper and access to the internet. As I said right at the beginning of this book, my aim is to help you to feel more positive and prepared for life with two children – to gently nudge you towards feelings of excitement, rather than worry. But, for now, it's OK to be worried so don't rush yourself to sort out everything, especially your emotions, too soon.

Concerns about your mental health during pregnancy

Although a wide range of emotions is to be expected in a second pregnancy, there are certain mental-health issues that can occur that necessitate extra help – specifically, antenatal anxiety and depression. Many people are familiar with post-natal depression, but few are aware that depression can also affect women *during* pregnancy. Antenatal anxiety is another condition that can affect women during pregnancy and its occurrence is similar to that of antenatal depression, with both affecting between seven and twenty per cent of mothers-to-be.[1] It's also possible that any mental-health issues that affected you at a previous point in your life can resurface or worsen during pregnancy.

Can mental-health issues develop in a second pregnancy, if there weren't any the first time?

The short answer is yes. Triggers for mental-health issues are different for everybody. If you find yourself struggling at any point, it is always worth discussing your feelings with a health-care professional. They can let you know if they think that what you're feeling is a little out of the ordinary and help you to access the proper treatment. You should seek advice if you recognise any of the following:

Symptoms of antenatal depression

- Severe lack of energy and feelings of exhaustion

- Tearfulness and crying a lot

- Feeling isolated and detached from others

- Being fearful of being judged by others

- Feeling overwhelmed and unable to cope like you usually do

- Issues with sleeping (not because of your child or pregnancy discomfort)

- Changes in your appetite beyond the usual expected in pregnancy

- Extreme levels of guilt

Symptoms of antenatal anxiety

- Extreme levels of anxiety about the pregnancy, new baby or firstborn child

- Panic attacks

- Feeling constantly on edge

- Physical symptoms of anxiety, such as tightness and tension

- Feelings of restlessness

- Increased levels of irritability

- Extremely anxious and distressing dreams and nightmares

If there were mental-health issues the first time around, will this happen again?

If you experienced mental-health issues during or after your first pregnancy, research suggests that you may be at an increased risk of developing them again.[2] This is by no means guaranteed, however, and you may have a very different experience the second time.

Finding support

Unless you already have specific contacts from your first pregnancy, your GP, midwife or health visitor (if you are still seeing one for your firstborn) will be the first point of call if you are worried about your mental health. They will be able to talk to you about your feelings and advise if they think any treatment and special care is necessary. They may refer you to a specialist counsellor, psychiatrist, psychologist, consultant or psychiatric nurse or, often, a mix of professionals. This team will help to reach a diagnosis and a treatment-and-support plan for you.

If you suffered with mental-health issues the first time around, it is important that you seek support as early as possible in your second pregnancy, even if you don't feel that you need it yet. Ideally, you would seek help beforehand – something known as pre-conception counselling. Building a support network early on means that professionals can keep an eye on your mental health and put any treatment plans into place, including those which may reduce the risk of recurrence, thus giving you the most positive experience of pregnancy.

As Sarah's story below shows, getting support as early as possible is important and ultimately beneficial to the whole family.

Sarah's story

My pregnancy with our first baby was magical. Though my husband and I weren't ready for baby number two until our son was over two, I yearned for and anticipated that maternal glow again. My expectations for pregnancy were high, so it was a surprise and a shock when all I felt during the first trimester of my second pregnancy was intense sadness, guilt and exhaustion. I was constantly tearful and couldn't believe that I was 'doing this' to my son. As we revealed the good news about becoming a big brother to our son, I sat crying while my husband smiled and told him how great this was. Luckily, he was excited, but his happy reaction didn't erase my fears and sadness; when intrusive thoughts occupied my mind, I finally realised that what I was experiencing was beyond the normal fears that accompany subsequent pregnancies – this was prenatal depression.

As a social worker and postpartum doula I knew all the signs, but it took me a while to see it when I was living it. I work for an organisation that supports women with PMADs (perinatal mood and anxiety disorders), so I quickly got in touch with a skilled therapist who also had extensive training in hormonal balance. Talking openly and honestly about my feelings helped remove the guilt I felt and took the power away from the thoughts. My therapist was able to help me see the significance of all the changes that happened in a short period of time and helped me recognise the physiological 'perfect storm' that contributed to my emotional instability: because of my reproductive history, I had been put on progesterone by my fertility endocrinologist just prior to discovering that I was pregnant again; the prescription, combined with the hormonal shift that accompanies weaning from breastfeeding (even when the cycle has returned, as mine had a year prior) left me physically sick, emotionally unstable and even more exhausted than is usual in the first trimester.

With proper treatment, I felt better emotionally at the start of my second trimester. I talked openly to my care team (acupuncturist, therapist, midwives, reproductive endocrinologist, birth and postpartum doulas) and planned early on for extensive help in the postpartum period as there is a greater likelihood of postpartum mood and anxiety disorders if a mum experiences issues prenatally. Though the pregnancy was tough, with the challenges of wrangling a toddler amid the tiredness that accompanies creating life, it forced me to slow down and make space for this new little being. Reframing the suffering and having professional support were key to my wellness. Unlike my expectations for pregnancy, I kept my expectations for life with two little ones very low, and have been pleasantly surprised by how rewarding it is. The theme of self-care is even more important now and I continue to outsource what I need to feel my best. It takes a village – for both pregnancy and parenting!

Rainbow babies

So far, we have only looked at families whose firstborn children are still living. For some of you, this sadly may not be the case and your current pregnancy may be a 'rainbow baby' (a baby born after a previous loss). In this situation, there are many elements of first-baby books that won't apply: while your firstborn may no longer be with you, there is no doubt that you are a second-time mother. For this reason, a lot of the thoughts and feelings you are having will be like those who have a living child. Feelings of guilt, concerns over replacing your lost baby with this new one, not remembering them as much while the new pregnancy takes up your headspace and worries about giving birth again are not the sorts of things you read about in most pregnancy and birth books aimed at first-timers. Similarly, as this is your second pregnancy and second birth, your body will also have changed.

The absolute key here is to find and accept emotional help as soon as possible. Get in touch with support organisations who can help to expertly guide you through the emotional roller-coaster that you will find yourself on (see Resources, page 268). Try speaking to others who have been in a similar position, through internet discussion forums and social-media groups. Again, you will find a list of these in the Resources section.

I am hugely grateful to the following mum for sharing her story, and that of her firstborn and her rainbow baby (to protect the family's privacy, I've simply given the initials of their first names).

E's story

My first pregnancy ended with the unexplained stillbirth of our daughter, E. Our world was totally blown apart and we weren't sure if we would ever recover from what we knew would be a lifelong grief, let alone be able to try for another child. Our arms were unbearably empty. However, we had always talked about wanting to have more than one child, so after receiving some reassurance that there was no known medical reason why we should suffer the loss of another baby, we felt we owed it to her to try and give her a living sibling. We found ourselves pregnant again less than six months after she'd died. The morning I got a positive pregnancy test I happened to have already scheduled placing the memorial marker at E's grave and I was experiencing a surreal mix of immense joy and deep sadness.

I don't think either of us quite anticipated the emotional rollercoaster of a journey we were about to embark upon, and to say we were disappointed by the lack of understanding and compassion shown to us by many medical professionals, as well as some family and friends, would be an understatement. We muddled through the pregnancy, shed a lot of anxious tears, and counted a lot of kicks (as reassurance that our baby was still alive), nervously counting down the days until my delivery date. The charities Sands, JOEL: The Complete Package and Tommy's were all absolute lifelines and I reached out to them all at one point or another.

After what felt like an incredibly long time, we were finally heading to the hospital to get labour started. I'd always been an advocate of natural births, but no longer trusted my body to keep our baby safe, so went with the medical advice to induce a week before the point at which our firstborn had died, so he would only just be classed as full term. We prepared for a stay in NICU in case our son had any problems breathing, but really our focus was on getting him out alive; our attitude was that we would deal with any issues caused by a slightly premature eviction as and when we needed to. The delivery was incredibly stressful, but he emerged crying, which was the biggest relief, and coped just fine breathing on his own straight away, so it wasn't long before we were able to head home.

I don't think either of us had let ourselves get our hopes up too high that we would actually be bringing him home, so we felt spectacularly unprepared to parent a living child, both physically and emotionally. We were already mentally exhausted after coping with the stress of the pregnancy and he was not a brilliant sleeper, so that really took its toll. I doubted my instincts on a great many things because of the guilt and grief I was dealing with over my daughter's death and found myself scouring the library and internet for help from those more experienced and expert than myself, as I was desperate to do things 'right' and not let anyone down again.

Parenting a second baby after losing your first can be incredibly daunting and extremely hard work, partly because I think many people don't realise that you are still a parent to two babies – it's just that you can't see one of them. I had to remind myself that no longer having the headspace or physical resources to devote every waking moment I had to honouring our daughter was not in any way a betrayal. It was completely normal and natural to feel torn in different directions when having another child, and she would understand why I couldn't visit her grave as regularly. I also had to remind myself that I was still grieving though, and allowing those feelings of sadness and longing to coexist alongside the gratitude and happiness I was now able to enjoy was an important part of adjusting to life as a mother of two. I also had to find other ways to connect with bereaved families and safe places to share my grief, so that it didn't get too much to bottle up and deal with alone.

Attending 'normal' playgroups was fairly excruciating at times because I had to have a carefully rehearsed series of lines prepared for the all-too-common, 'Is-this-your-first-baby?' question. But the temptation to retreat from the world was thankfully outweighed by my need to get out and about among other human beings; my son J and I did not do each other any favours through, being cooped up indoors all day, and I wouldn't have met some lovely, supportive people who I now count as dear friends had I not been brave enough to venture out.

Connecting with other bereaved parents who understand more than most what a bittersweet reality this can be even in seemingly the most mundane of moments has been an essential part of me staying sane. And appreciating that I am not – and never will be – a perfect parent is a work in progress, because I am forever trying to make it up to my daughter and prove to her that I do deserve to raise her living siblings.

What might be different second time around?

Second pregnancies tend to be different to first ones in many ways and, of course, all pregnancies are different in any case. It's therefore hard to provide a definitive list of what may be different this time around, but here are some of the most common points.

- **Time flies** With your first pregnancy you probably knew exactly how big your baby was at any given point and what fruit or vegetable their size compared to. And when people asked how far gone you were, you could doubtless reply with the exact number of weeks and days. This time, busy with another child to look after, you may struggle to remember how many weeks you are and have very little idea about the size of your baby, much less have time to fill in a pregnancy journal every week. This can often leave you feeling guilty, for focusing less on number two than number one. But on the plus side, the pregnancy tends to fly by!

- **Less focus on birth and more on afterwards** When you're pregnant for the first time it's hard to really think about life after the birth. When I taught antenatal classes, it was always difficult to get first-time parents-to-be to think about life with a newborn; they were so focused on giving birth that they didn't have any headspace to devote new parenthood. The second time around, this is often flipped on its head, with second-time parents being more focused on life once the new baby arrives and preparing their firstborn for the arrival of a sibling. It's still important to think about the birth though, which is why I have devoted a whole chapter to it (see Chapter 6).

- **Fewer new friends** You're less likely to make new friends who are at the same stage of pregnancy as you. The first time around, you may well have gone to ante-natal classes, or meet-ups afterwards with parents of similar-aged babies. This time, you will probably keep the parent friends that you already have.

- **More tiredness** Combine the lack of opportunity to rest, the physical demands of looking after a busy young child, the sleepless nights that often accompany the tiring days and the exhaustion that new pregnancy brings and it's likely you will feel more tired this time.

- **Sensitive breasts** Breast sensitivity is common in pregnancy, particularly in the first trimester as your body adjusts to the hormonal changes. If you are still breastfeeding your firstborn, however, you may find that they become significantly more sensitive. Some mums find that they need to restrict or limit feeds until this sensation passes, others feel that they need to stop breastfeeding, though many continue. I will discuss tandem feeding (breastfeeding both the new baby and your firstborn) more in the next chapter.

- **Bump size** Most mums 'show' quicker with their second pregnancy and their bump will probably be bigger. In part, this is because your body has already stretched after the birth of your first baby and you may also be slightly heavier yourself. Research has also shown that second babies are, on average, 138g bigger than first babies.[3]

- **Diastasis recti** After the birth of your first baby, your abdominal muscles may not have returned to normal, leaving a gap between the two sides of the rectus abdominis muscle. Known as diastasis recti, this separation causes weakened abdominal muscles and can lead to back pain. If you suspect this is an issue for you, then either a personal trainer qualified in working with pregnant mums or a physiotherapist can help with specific exercises.

- **Weaker pelvic floor** Your first pregnancy and birth are likely to have impacted on your pelvic-floor strength and you may find that it is weaker during your second pregnancy, leading to a degree of bladder incontinence. If you don't feel that pelvic-floor exercises are working for you, speak to your midwife or GP about alternative options.

- **Braxton Hicks** Although you would have experienced Braxton Hicks (or 'practice') contractions with your first baby, you may well find that you notice them more and experience them more strongly in your second pregnancy. They are also likely to start earlier than they did the first time around.

- **Shorter pregnancy** Research has shown that second pregnancies are an average of five days shorter than first ones.[4]

- **Less frequent midwife appointments** If your first pregnancy and birth were uncomplicated, you will probably need fewer midwife appointments second time around because you are less liable to develop complications. Mums-to-be who are pregnant for the first time usually have around ten appointments with their midwife or doctor, whereas second-time mums usually have around seven.

- **No antenatal or pregnancy classes** For a first pregnancy, most parents-to-be attend antenatal preparation classes of some form and many attend pregnancy exercise classes. Second time around, there is obviously less time for these, as well as childcare to consider. You're also unlikely to be invited to NHS birth preparation courses. I genuinely believe, however, that both are hugely beneficial second time around, and I will talk a little more about this in Chapter 6, when looking at second births.

- **Less help** When you're pregnant with your second child, people are often not as forthcoming with help as they were the first time. They seem to think that because you're an 'old hand' at this now, you don't need help. Ironically, however, your second pregnancy is probably when you need the most help. While the lack of fuss and constant questioning may be welcome, it can also leave you feeling a little overlooked and uncared for. See page 70 for more about the importance of asking for help.

Coping with physical symptoms

Morning sickness and tiredness, when you're pregnant with your first child often come as a nasty shock, especially in the first trimester. Many first-time mums-to-be have to cope with early pregnancy and work at a stage when most keep their pregnancies secret. The biggest plus about pregnancy as a first-timer, however, is being able to fully relax when you are home. I had awful nausea and pelvic pain in my first pregnancy and while the days at work were hard, I used to come home in the evening and relax. At weekends I would have long lie-ins, lazy days and many naps.

Second time around, however, I was awake by six o'clock every morning, inevitably had a toddler clinging to my legs every time I visited the bathroom when the nausea turned into vomiting and, despite the fact that my son still napped every day, my house was such a devastation zone that I felt I had to spend his naptimes cooking, cleaning and trying to get on top of an ever-growing laundry pile. If I ever did manage to nap, my son would wake and cry for me just as I had dozed off. Although I didn't return to work after my maternity leave ended, I was well and truly exhausted, and I remember often wondering why I thought it was hard the first time around.

As my pregnancy progressed, I realised that I had to take control and schedule in some rest time. With no family on hand, we had two options: ask for help from friends or pay for it. We did both. A friend and I each took care of the other's children once or twice a month, to give the other one time to rest, shop or just catch up on things. We were also lucky enough to be able to afford a childminder for one morning a week. The first time my son went to the childminder, I frantically spent all the time cleaning. I didn't make that mistake again, and the next week I slept for almost the whole time he was there. In the following weeks, I either slept or rested. My standards around the house dropped dramatically and I stopped trying to take over my partner's attempts at house-work. (I'm a bit of a perfectionist and tended to redo whatever he did!) When the washing pile became overwhelming we dropped some off at our local launderette and got it service washed. The washing came back clean and folded, ready to put away, and at very little cost. When it came to eating, we had more takeaways and ready meals than I'd care to admit. And when my pelvic pain and sickness were at their worst, my husband used to pack up a little picnic bag for us full of food for the day. This meant I could give my son lunch without having to move very much.

If my son napped, I took the opportunity to rest, sleep or listen to a pregnancy relaxation recording. I had to really fight the urge to get up and do more around the house. I told myself time and time again, 'The house can wait, but you need to rest – for the baby as much as you'. It took me a long time to stop feeling guilty. I also came up with ways to entertain my son that didn't involve much movement or effort from me, on the days when my husband was at work. These included:

- water painting (a paintbrush and bowl of water) on the patio, while I lay on a sunbed alongside (he could do this for hours)

- drawing on my legs with lip- and eyeliner, while I lay down on the bed or sofa

- rice sensory play – a large plastic container of uncooked rice (sometimes dyed with food colouring) with different plastic animals, metal cars and sand toys to play with

- water play in a warm bath together with lots of bubbles and bath toys; in the warmer weather we did the same in a big paddling pool in the garden

- watching TV – I'm not a great fan of screen time, but I'm more of a believer in 'do the least harm', and sometimes TV was the only thing that got us through the day; on days when I felt really bad, we spent many hours cuddling and watching TV together.

I spoke to mums about how they felt during their second pregnancies and what tips they would give others in the same situation. Here are some of their replies:

My second pregnancy was so tiring, I made sure to nap with my toddler when I could, drank lots of water and ate little and often. On the plus side, it went so quickly because of having a small one-year-old to run around after.

You cope because you have to. I used some of my annual leave to have days off when number one was at nursery, so that I had time to rest.

I was so tired with my second pregnancy, that I started going to bed at 8pm, right after my daughter. I also showered with her at night, before bedtime, so there was a bit less rushing in the mornings, but also because it was such a nice bonding moment – just us – before a new baby was going to literally be in between the two of us.

My advice is to take the help people offer. Neither you nor your child benefits from an exhausted mum.

If you can, try to have midwife appointments at your own home.

I had bad hyperemesis gravidarum [a severe form of pregnancy sickness] with lots of hospital admissions and accompanying exhaustion, but my partner's work was flexible. Thankfully, my eldest had a great relationship with my mother who was twenty minutes away. We somehow just managed.

Finding help

As you'll see from most of these quotes, and my own experiences, finding and accepting help is key to surviving pregnancy when you already have a young child. If you have family within a reasonable distance who haven't come forward yet, then you should approach them. Tell them that you would really appreciate them taking care of your firstborn for a couple of hours, so you can rest. And if this goes well, ask if it's something they could consider doing regularly.

If your relatives don't live near by or are not happy to help, the following are all possible alternatives:

- **Doulas** While most people associate doulas with birth (see Chapter 6), they can also be invaluable when you are pregnant. Many are happy to come and help with housework, cooking and entertaining older siblings. Doulas who are still training offer a reduced fee and can be a good alternative to a fully qualified doula (remember, most trainee doulas are still experienced mothers). You may also be entitled to financial help through certain access funds, such as that offered by Doula UK, which enables those on a low income to receive free or reduced-fee doula services.

- **Childminders** A childminder can be useful for giving you a few child-free hours to relax. Not all childminders offer part-time slots, or ad-hoc care, but many do. They are usually cheaper than doulas.

- **Mother's helps** Mother's helps are generally self-employed, freelance workers, but they can also work for agencies. They help with anything from household admin to shopping and childcare.

- **Students** People studying childcare, teaching, midwifery and the like at college and university can be a great source of help, with their knowledge and (often) first-aid training. Many will be searching for work over academic holidays. Contacting local colleges, sixth-form centres and universities or local mummy groups on social media can often prove fruitful.

- **Babysitting circle with other mums** If you have a group of mum friends, perhaps from antenatal classes first time around, you could suggest setting up a babysitting circle, swapping childcare with another family.

- **Support charities** Depending on where you live and your circumstances, there may be free help available from local charities, such as Home-Start. These organisations can provide volunteer help, offering emotional support and playing with older children while you rest a little.

You will find a list of different organisations who may be able to offer help in the Resources.

Your toddler vs your bump

One of the top worries of second-time mums-to-be is protecting their growing baby from a rambunctious toddler or preschooler. I remember being out shopping with my firstborn when he ran headlong into my bump, so hard he winded me. Convinced that he'd done some serious harm, I rang my midwife who managed to calm me down, telling me that everything would be fine.

Growing babies are cushioned in the waters of the amniotic sac and surrounded by layers of muscle, fat and skin, so they are well protected. What matters more is how *you* feel about your bump being climbed, sat and bounced on. Towards the end of my pregnancy, my skin felt very tight and sore and my hips were almost constantly achy. No longer worried about my baby, I had to discourage my firstborn's 'bump bouncing' for my own benefit. I worked hard to get him to lay alongside, rather than on top of me whenever we cuddled, and every time he tried to bounce, I calmly lifted him up, sat him next to me and said, 'Stop. That hurts.' If he cried, which he did the first few times, I gave him a big hug and said, 'It's OK. I'm not mad at you. I just can't let you do that because it hurts me.' He was only little, and I have no idea if he really understood (I doubt it, to be honest); however, what he did understand was that bump bouncing was now strictly off the menu. Staying calm and – most importantly – consistent when implementing and upholding the 'no-bouncing' boundary is the key to stopping the unwanted behaviour. Don't get angry though, and be ready to comfort with lots of hugs, kisses and reassurance if your child gets upset. It may take several weeks before your child gets the message, but in time they will, and the bump bouncing should stop. If, however, you are not uncomfortable with it, there is no reason to stop it out of concern for your baby's safety.

Tricky behaviour from your firstborn during your pregnancy

Most advice regarding a firstborn's challenging behaviour tends to focus on after the new baby has arrived (see Chapter 10 for more on this). However, this isn't the only time their behaviour may deteriorate – it's also very common to see changes during your pregnancy, particularly in the third trimester. Children may become withdrawn, sulk, whine more and shun affection from their mums during later pregnancy. Or they may show completely the opposite behaviour and become much more clingy and needy, not wanting to be separated from their mums, whether that manifests in difficult drop-offs or flat-out refusal to go to preschool or nursery in the daytime or no longer being happy with Dad putting them to bed at night. Sometimes they can become destructive or defiant. They may also regress in potty training, having accidents when they have been previously dry, or during sleep, with many more night wakings.

So why might firstborns struggle during pregnancy?

- They receive less attention from parents and friends and relatives who are focusing on the impending new arrival.

- Mums become less able to do things with them, particularly playing, as they get bigger and have less energy.

- If a mum has severe sickness, tiredness, pain, discomfort, or if she is hospitalised during pregnancy, they can feel less connected to her – not just physically, but emotionally too.

- They may feel that change is coming, but not truly understand it, and struggle to cope with the uncertainty.

- Lots of physical changes may be happening in their lives – they may be moving to a new house, swapping bedrooms, moving to a bed from a cot, starting preschool or nursery, sorting out their old toys and equipment ... Change is rarely met well by toddlers and preschoolers.

- They may be scared by medical appointments, such as hospital visits, ultrasound scans, blood tests and bump palpating (feeling for baby's size and position).

The best advice I can give you is that almost any behaviour your child displays during your pregnancy is normal and it won't last for ever. This is a big transition for you and your partner and it's a huge transition for your firstborn. Just as you may feel anxiety, doubt, confusion and fear about what's going to happen to your little family over the coming months, your firstborn may well feel the same. And that's OK. These feelings, like yours, can be worked with. It's possible to allay their fears, remove confusion and prepare them in a positive way for what's to come – which is exactly what I'll discuss in the next chapter. For now, the most important thing you can do is to empathise with your child. Understand that they are not behaving in this way to be difficult or to deliberately annoy you. Keep reminding yourself that they are only a child and having a new baby brother or sister is a big thing to them. It's natural and normal to have hiccups during pregnancy, when that new sibling is so intangible to them. Your role is to explain, reassure and connect as much as you can. But how do you do that – especially when you're exhausted, feeling poorly or maybe even in hospital? You talk, you cuddle and you 'hold' your child metaphorically. You allow them to feel what they're feeling – to cry, to vent their anger and confusion – and you meet their big feelings as much as you can with patience, love and support, whether that's at bedtime, with a fifteen-minute cuddle on the sofa or during visiting hours. Combine this with some of the preparation in the next chapter and a good dose of being kind to yourself – something we'll often come back to later in the book, when we look at feeling guilty ourselves.

Next, I'm going to outline some practical and emotional preparations that can really help the whole family.

Chapter 4

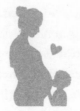

Preparing Number One for Number Two

M any second-time parents strike lucky with the transition to two children. They have 'easy babies' and their firstborns seem to take everything in their stride. You could be one of those lucky ones. But why leave to chance the future happiness of your growing family, when you can dramatically increase the odds in your favour with a healthy dose of preparation? The more you can prepare your home, your lifestyle, your routines, your expectations and, of course, your firstborn for the arrival of baby number two, the easier the transition will be. This chapter focuses on exactly that.

We'll begin by looking at some of the practical preparations that ideally should occur before your new baby arrives.

Practical preparations

Many of the practical preparations you can make in advance of your new baby's arrival are actually for your benefit as parents, rather than that of the baby or your older child. That doesn't mean it is somehow wrong to do them. I know many parents who worry about changing anything in their firstborn's life, not wanting to upset their equilibrium, and sacrificing their own energy and sometimes sanity as a result. But let's get this out there right now: it's OK to want to make life easier for yourself. In fact, the more you can prepare now to reduce work for yourself once the new baby arrives, the better in my book. The added bonus is that you should be more relaxed and calmer as a result, which means you'll be far less likely to lose your temper with your firstborn. So they will benefit too!

When should you start?

The only proviso regarding practical preparations is that you should make them as early as possible before your new baby's arrival. (One exception to this is potty training, which I discuss on page 90.) If I could summon up an ideal point by which you would not make any further changes, it would be somewhere in the sixth month of pregnancy, or around the beginning of the third trimester. Any later than this and there is a chance that your firstborn could link the changes to the new baby arriving and therefore struggle with them emotionally. You absolutely don't want your older child to feel pushed out to make way for the new arrival. What you need – or should I say, what your child needs – in the run-up to the baby arriving is stability. Stability and consistency are reassuring to young children, and at a time when almost everything else in their world is going to change, that matters more than ever.

Does this mean you should never change anything in the last trimester of pregnancy? Well, sometimes, it can't be helped. Moving to a new house is a great example; and potty training is another. Sometimes you must grasp the opportunities when they present and seize the moment, even if that moment is inconvenient. So if you must make changes late in your pregnancy, please don't worry too much. Just try to make the bulk of them as early on as possible.

Do you *have* to change anything?

No, you don't. As I mentioned above, some families luck out. They don't prepare anything and everything slots into place. And some families cope better with unpredictability than others; some even thrive on it. If you are happy with how things are now, and you don't feel the need to change anything – at least not yet, anyway, then don't. What matters most is that you're comfortable with how things are. If you think you'd rather 'suck it and see', then skip this section and go straight to Emotional Preparations, page 91.

Sorting out your firstborn's sleep

Whether your firstborn is sleeping through the night or waking every hour, putting some steps in place now to improve their sleep and providing triggers that can help them to feel relaxed at night in your absence, is a key part of the 'calm second-time parents' puzzle.

Here are the top five sleep changes that second-time parents-to-be commonly focus on:

1. Reducing night wakings

This is almost always at the top of the list of things to change when it comes to sleep. If your firstborn still wakes regularly at night, it makes sense to gently encourage them to sleep a little more solidly before introducing a new baby, who will need you lots at night. Night waking is a big part of early childhood and remains so until around the age of four years.

Night wakings in the toddler and preschool years tend to have emotional rather than physical causes. Nightmares, night terrors, fear of the dark and things that lurk in it and separation anxiety all feature highly. Making sure your child has a good nightlight on all night can really help, as can the introduction of a special bedtime buddy – a toy you choose together that your child is tasked to look after at night. Explain to your child that their bedtime buddy might get scared or lonely at night, and that if that happens, they need to give him or her a big hug and make sure they're OK. This works by transferring the child's anxieties onto the bedtime buddy and is much more effective than telling the child to hug the toy if they feel scared themselves.

In terms of lighting, your child should only be exposed to light on the red spectrum at night. White, blue, green, pink, purple or yellow light can inhibit the secretion of melatonin, the sleep hormone, whereas red has no negative impact on it.[1] Light also matters in the run-up to bedtime. For the best sleep, children should not be exposed to screens (televisions, tablets or phones) in the two hours before bedtime and any lighting around them should be dim, including that in the bathroom.[2]

Introducing a bedtime snack just before the bedtime routine starts can also be helpful, especially if you include food that contains tryptophan (an amino acid that aids production of melatonin) and magnesium (a mineral that aids relaxation). Good choices are wholemeal bread, perhaps toasted, with almond butter, or porridge oats with slices of banana.

Naps impact a lot on night sleep in the toddler and preschool years. Research has shown that napping in the day after two years of age can have a negative impact on night sleep, and although it can give you much needed time to rest and relax during pregnancy, sometimes it comes at the expense of a better night's sleep.[3]

Finally, the actual timing of bedtime matters too. Research has shown that toddlers and preschoolers are chemically ready to sleep at around eight o'clock at night.[4] This is when their bodies have secreted sufficient melatonin for restful sleep. Aiming for an earlier bedtime can be counterproductive if your child resists it, as it can result in a more drawn-out bedtime and more night waking.

2. Reducing Mum-centred bedtimes

I work with many second-time mothers-to-be who are anxious about settling their firstborns to sleep once the new baby arrives. They may be breastfeeding and worried about others getting their child to sleep, or they may simply have a child who has a strong preference for their company at bedtime over anyone else. Whatever the reason, their goal is the same – to encourage their child to accept somebody else settling them to sleep.

The best way to achieve this is to involve the other parent or a family member in bedtime as much as possible, and for as long as possible, before the new baby arrives. This doesn't have to be the actual getting to sleep; it could be bath time, story time, getting changed into pyjamas and so on. The more the other person does, the better. This means that the child will be used to them being around at bedtime, which means it's not such a huge change if Mum can't be there in the future.

The other thing you need to do is to really work on the bond between the child and the other adult in the daytime. Lots and lots of play and shared activities are key – for instance, going swimming together (without Mum) every Saturday morning or going to the park together (without Mum) every Sunday afternoon. The unexpected benefit here is that this extra 'Mum-free' time gives you the chance to catch up on some sleep during pregnancy, or in the early postnatal days.

Unfortunately, there is no secret in getting children to accept comfort from somebody else at bedtime, even once you have involved the other adult(s) in bedtime and worked hard on their relationship during the daytime. It simply takes lots of time and patience. I always tell parents that the best thing to do is to reset their expectations of what settling without Mum at bedtime will look like. It's unlikely that it will ever be as calm and relaxed (or quick) as when she does it. There will be crying. (Initially there may be a lot of crying.) In time, however, this will lessen and eventually stop. The adult's aim in trying to settle the child shouldn't be to replicate bedtime with Mum, without tears. Instead, they should aim to stay calm and patient and comfort the child while they cry. Research has shown that when children cry, but are offered comfort by a caring adult, their bodies do not release the same amount of the stress hormone cortisol as when they are crying alone.[5] So whoever is settling can rest assured that even if the child is crying in Mum's absence, that is OK, so long as they are responsive and give lots of cuddles. In other words, don't fear crying, but never leave the child to cry alone.

3. Vacating the cot and changing bedrooms

If your firstborn currently sleeps in a cot, with a sleep positioner or cushion that you'd like to use for the new baby, or you'd like to move them to a new room, then as with all changes, the earlier you make the move to the new sleep setup the better. Ideally, you want your older child used to their new bed and room for several months before the new baby arrives – not just because you don't want them to feel pushed out by the new baby's arrival but because any changes in sleep invariably cause regressions of some sort. When you first transition a toddler out of a cot and into a bed for instance, it's the first time they have the freedom to get up and explore in the night – and they tend to make the most of it! This regression is only temporary and usually passes on its own, in time, without any input from you.

4. Ending bedsharing – or preparing to bedshare with both children

If you want to end bedsharing with your first child before the new baby arrives then, much like moving bedrooms or changing from a cot to a bed, it's important that your firstborn doesn't feel they have been evicted from your bed to make way for the new arrival. Of course, in a way, this is exactly what has happened, but if the older child senses this, you are likely to be faced with a lot of upset and sleepless nights when the baby arrives. I always recommend that you stop bedsharing by the sixth month of pregnancy, or, if you don't quite make it by then, wait until the baby is at least three months old to make the change. By this point, hopefully, the firstborn will have got over the initial stages of the big sibling transition and will fare better with ending bedsharing. Stopping between the sixth month of pregnancy and three months postnatal almost never ends well though.

You could set up a toddler bed or a single mattress on the floor in your bedroom if space allows, so that your firstborn will still feel close to you in the same room, but you will have space for the new baby in your bed. Again, if you make this change, I'd recommend you do it at least three months before the new baby arrives.

Of course, you don't have to end bedsharing just because a new baby is joining the family. Around the world, many families share their beds, or their bedrooms, with many children. If you'd like to continue bedsharing, then the only change you'll need to make is in terms of positioning. There should always be at least one adult in between the baby and older sibling, or preferably two. This prevents the older child from accidentally climbing onto, or rolling on, the baby in the night. This means that with the new baby on the outside of the bed, next to you, the ideal place for the older child is on the other side of the bed, next to your partner (see diagram).

If you think that you may want to bedshare with both children and your budget and bedroom size allow, upgrading your current bed to a king-size or super-king (basically, the biggest bed that you can afford and will fit in your bedroom) is a great investment. Creating a family bed, that can be used for many years to come, is a great way to meet everybody's needs and get a little more sleep.

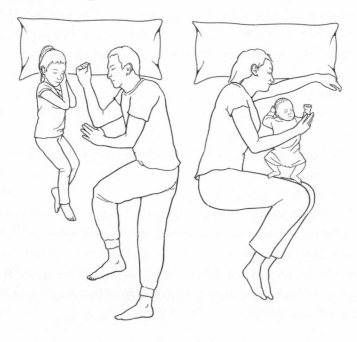

5. A future-proof bedtime routine

As with reducing reliance on Mum at bedtime, 'future-proofing' your older child's bedtime routine to allow for the new baby's needs can be incredibly helpful. By this, I mean think about what you might do at bedtime when the new baby arrives. Do you have a partner who gets home at seven o'clock? If so, nudging the start of bedtime to after this time will be a huge help. This means that your partner can watch the baby while you put your firstborn to bed, or can take charge of bedtime if the baby needs you. If you're a single parent, or your partner works late or is often away, focusing on creating a little more independence at bedtime can help. For instance, you could try introducing bedtime story audiobooks or mindfulness relaxation recordings for your child to fall asleep to at bedtime, which will allow you to tuck them up and then return to the baby, if necessary. You could also think about moving bath time to first thing in the morning, removing the need to juggle bath time with a newborn and older child. The more you can structure your firstborn's bedtime routine to accommodate the needs of a baby (who despite the best-laid plans will always need settling unexpectedly!) before their arrival, the easier the transition will be.

Weaning from breastfeeding

If you're currently breastfeeding your firstborn, you may be worried about what will happen when the new baby arrives. Perhaps you hope to tandem feed (that is, to breastfeed both the new baby and your firstborn), or perhaps you hope to stop breastfeeding before the birth. There are certainly pros and cons for both, but ultimately, this is a personal decision. You need to do what you feel is best for you and your family. I've worked with many families who successfully tandem feed and feel that it is the best decision they could have made, for their firstborn and themselves. I've also helped mums to stop breastfeeding, because they felt they really wanted to do so before the new baby arrived, allowing them to focus solely on the baby.

But before we talk about weaning, let's take a closer look at tandem feeding.

Breastfeeding throughout pregnancy and tandem feeding

Continuing breastfeeding throughout the new pregnancy, and sometimes afterwards, can provide a much gentler transition for a firstborn child. Unfortunately, there are many myths surrounding this, the most common of which relate to safety – that is, the safety of the pregnancy and the potential impact of breastfeeding on miscarriage, premature birth and the growth and development of the new baby. These concerns are all unfounded. Research has found no statistically significant risk of miscarriage in pregnancies where the mother was breastfeeding another child, compared to those where the mother had already ceased breastfeeding.[6] Further studies comparing pregnancy outcomes of mothers who continued to breastfeed an older child throughout their pregnancy with those who did not, found no difference between the two groups.[7] There were no more premature births or low birth weights for mothers who breastfed throughout pregnancy than for those who did not. Simply put, breastfeeding will not harm the new pregnancy or baby. But it could really help your firstborn.

What about after the birth? Will the new baby get enough milk if your toddler or preschooler is still breastfeeding? The general school of thought is that it is important for the newborn to feed first in the first few days after birth, to ensure that they get sufficient quantities of colostrum, the first milk, which is much needed for the development of the immune system and gut bacteria of the new baby. As colostrum is in limited supply, the new baby needs to have priority over their older sibling initially. Once the first few postnatal days have passed, you will probably have more than enough milk for both children. The simplest approach is to keep a close eye on your newborn, and make sure that they are displaying signs of getting enough milk (frequent wet and dirty nappies). If they are thriving, then there is no need to restrict your older child's feeds or to make sure the newborn feeds first.

While feeding throughout pregnancy and tandem nursing work brilliantly for some mothers, others strongly feel that they wish to stop breastfeeding before their baby's birth. My advice, as always, is that any big changes happen well in advance of the new baby's arrival, so if you want to wean your toddler or preschooler, it is best to do so by the time you are six months pregnant. This means that enough time will have passed between weaning and the new baby arriving for your older child to be settled with the idea, and it is far less likely to result in turmoil or in your older child wanting to start breastfeeding again when they see their new sibling doing so.

When it comes to weaning, you have different options, ranging from weaning completely to just dropping the night feeds and potentially restricting day feeds. Again, there is no right or wrong, so simply do what works best for you.

How to night wean

Night weaning is usually the first step towards weaning breastfeeding, and it is what I would recommend starting with. If you wean from breastfeeding during the day first, you often find that the night feeds really ramp up because the child tries to make up for the feeds they haven't received in the daytime. Often, sleep regresses and things become much harder. Weaning the night feeds first, however, usually results in better sleep and doesn't seem to cause increased feeding in the daytime. You could go 'cold turkey' on night feeds, and instead of feeding, just offer your child lots of hugs, cuddles and reassurance – however, in my experience, this is usually very stressful for both you and the child. Instead, I advise a slightly slower approach, whereby you delay feeding at each waking a little more each night: instead of feeding, you offer as much comfort as you can for increasing lengths of time, before finally offering the breast. I suggest that – at least to start with – you always feed at bedtime. This feed is very important to most children, so I recommend leaving weaning from this one till last.

This is how the process looks (although timings can be flexible):

- **Night 1** Breastfeed at bedtime as usual (to sleep, or until the child has finished – either is fine); then every single time your child wakes, comfort them for five minutes (pick up, rock, pat, cuddle, stroke, sing, offer water and so on) and then breastfeed if it is obvious they are not going to settle without a feed.

- **Night 2** Exactly as above, but this time comfort for ten minutes, before breastfeeding if it is obvious they are not going to settle without it.

- **Night 3** As above, but comfort for fifteen minutes, then breastfeed if it is obvious they are not going to settle without it.

- **Night 4** As before, but with a twenty-minute delay at each waking.

- **Night 5** As before, but now with a twenty-five-minute delay.

- **Night 6 onwards** As before, but now with a thirty-minute delay at each waking. Keep the delay before breastfeeding at thirty minutes for all subsequent nights.

When you start the night-weaning process, you must be consistent and delay every time the child wakes. The worst thing you can do is to not delay at one waking once you've started. Delays can be handled by either parent; if there are two of you, then it's great to take turns, so that the onus is not only on one of you. The aim of this process is to help the child to realise that they can take comfort from something that isn't the breast. It's important that they are never left to cry alone; they should always be cuddled and comforted. Usually, you will see a big difference in night wakings by around Days 7–10 when following this process. It doesn't mean the child will sleep through but, hopefully, it will be easier and quicker to settle them back to sleep when they do wake, and they won't be reliant on breastfeeding to settle, meaning that either parent (and others) can help.

Weaning from breastfeeding completely

If you feel that you would like to wean from breastfeeding completely before your new baby arrives, then, as previously, the earlier in the pregnancy you start the better. The whole process of weaning from the breast gently takes a couple of months because it works at the child's pace as much as possible. The first step is to night wean, in the way I have just described. Once you have done this, you may find that your desire to stop breastfeeding in the day and at bedtime isn't as strong. If this is the case, then I would recommend waiting a month or so before any further weaning. If you decide that you are still keen to wean completely, then my advice is to work first on the feeds that are unrelated to sleep. So if your child still naps, aim to wean all daytime feeds apart from those given just before a nap and at bedtime. If your child no longer naps, then aim to wean all feeds except for the one at bedtime. As mentioned previously, the bedtime feed should be the very last to go; it's usually the most important feed to the child and trying to get them to sleep without it can be very hard, often resulting in much tougher and longer bedtimes. So do be very sure you want to stop it before you try, and be aware that bedtime could become much harder.

To wean in the daytime, first aim to 'never offer, but never refuse'. This means that for a couple of weeks at least, if your child requests a feed in the daytime, you always respond and allow them to feed, if possible. However, if they are not specifically asking for a feed, then don't ever offer. For instance, if they are grumpy and crying but not asking for a feed, offer hugs and verbal comfort where you would usually offer the breast. The only exception here is the bedtime feed, when you should offer it straight away.

Once 'never offer, but never refuse' is well established, the next step is to delay feeding in the daytime, in the same way as night weaning (see page 86). So on Day 1, try to delay feeding when they request it by offering alternative comfort for five minutes (and then feeding). The next day, increase this to ten minutes and so on, until you are delaying offering a feed for half an hour each time they ask for it. From Day 7 onwards, you may want to stop offering the breast completely and instead provide lots of hugs, comfort and verbal reassurance. Within two weeks, most children will have reduced breastfeeding to only the bedtime feed, which you can always continue to offer if you wish to keep it. If not, follow the same process to remove this feed too.

Starting day care or preschool

If your firstborn hasn't yet been away from you during the day and you are thinking about starting them in some form of day care or preschool, the earlier you start the transition the better. Any setting that your firstborn spends time in should be a known and reassuring constant to them by the time their new sibling arrives. To achieve this, they need to have attended for several months before the baby's arrival and have had time to really settle in, make friends and form a bond with their primary caregiver. This can be hard on you emotionally – lots of parents feel that they should be making the most of the last of their time alone with their firstborn and it can often feel wrong sending them away and losing some of that precious time. But remember – this really is in their best interests. The more settled and secure they are with their day-care or pre-school provider, the easier they will find the change when the new baby arrives. Think of the time that they are away from you as an opportunity to focus on the new baby and indeed, yourself, giving you the chance to prepare emotionally and physically and rest, so that when your child is back with you, you can concentrate on them with renewed energy.

If your child is already at day care or preschool, try to make sure that any changes there happen well before the new baby comes, the ideal being, again, no later than six months of pregnancy. These can include increasing hours at the setting, changing to a different one, changing keyworkers, or even changing rooms (for instance, moving up from the baby to the toddler room). If you can't work the changes by the sixth month of pregnancy, then it's best to wait until the new baby is at least three months old. Having a new sibling is all the change your older child needs to cope with for the first three months.

Potty training

I have mentioned many times that my ideal is to leave at least three months between making any changes and the new baby arriving. The only exception to this is potty training. Why? Because when children are ready, they're ready. Often, this is at the most inconvenient time: just before you go on holiday, just before you move to a new house and just before – or after – you have welcomed a new baby to the family. If you ignore your child's signs of potty-training readiness, there's a strong chance that it will be a lot harder when you decide you have time to devote to it. The very best time to potty train is when a child is ready, both emotionally and physically. If they are truly ready, the whole experience is usually quick, straight-forward and relatively easy. So while it may be inconvenient to potty train when you are eight months pregnant, it will be easier for all of you in the long run. In *The Gentle Potty Training Book*, I talk about signs of readiness, the main ones being that your child:

- is around twenty to thirty months old

- is dry and clean for at least three hours at a time

- often wakes from a nap, or in the morning, with a dry, clean nappy

- tells you that they need a pee or a poo before they do it

- resists wearing a nappy

- hides to poo

- can communicate their physical needs to you – for instance saying, 'I'm hungry' or 'I'm cold'

- can take down their own trousers (elasticated) and underwear

- asks to wear underwear

- asks to use the potty or toilet.

If you identify at least two, preferably three of these signs, then your child is ready to go. However pregnant you are, grab the chance and go for it!

Emotional preparations

It may surprise you but preparing your child practically for the arrival of number two is, in my opinion, probably the most important form of preparation. Many people believe that emotional preparation is more important, but the more you prepare the practical stuff, the more you are laying the groundwork for the emotional side of things. It's also harder to prepare young children fully in emotional terms, and to understand why this is we need to look at the development of different cognitive processes or, more specifically, abstract and hypothetical thinking.

Abstract thinking

Abstract thinking describes the thought processes required to understand that something exists, even when it's not tangible. Young children have poor abstract-thinking skills. A reception-aged child doing mathematics requires certain props – number stackers, counters or blocks – to help them with addition and subtraction. This need to touch something, to manipulate it, continues throughout the first few years at school. What the child is demonstrating here is an inability to manipulate and understand objects with just their mind, or in other words abstract thinking. Scientists believe that children develop a good working grasp of abstract thinking during adolescence; before this, their brain development means that they struggle to grasp abstract concepts.

Hypothetical thinking

Hypothetical thinking describes the thought processes required to understand the impact of things that haven't happened yet. In short, it's a little like predicting the future, but by applying logic. For instance, you may have a desire to throw a ball inside a china shop, but you know that it isn't a good idea because the ball will probably hit a fragile object and break it. Hypothetical thinking is a mature cognitive skill. Young children often cause accidents and break things because they simply don't – and can't – think through the consequences of their actions. And teenagers struggle with this, too, which is why so many of them do such stupid things!

If we think about the thought processes required to process the arrival of a new sibling, both abstract and hypothetical thinking play a huge role. To understand what is about to happen to them when a new baby arrives, children need to grasp the idea that the baby exists, even though they can't see it, other than in a blurry ultrasound image and, more importantly, they can't touch it. Secondly, to really grasp what will happen when the baby is born, they need to be able to think hypothetically. They need to understand what impact the baby might have and how it will affect them. Unfortunately, they can do neither of these things.

Does this mean that it is futile to try and do any emotional preparation? No, I don't think it is. It is worth explaining about the new baby and what will happen to your firstborn. The chances are that they will take something in. However, it's important to be realistic about how effective any emotional preparation will be. So many new second-time parents are shocked when the baby arrives and their firstborn struggles. They say, 'But, we prepared so well. We read books, we watched videos, we involved our firstborn at every step, so why is he struggling so much?' My best tip is not to overestimate your firstborn's ability to understand what a tremendous change is about to happen. In my experience, being realistic about the impact of your emotional preparatory work is so important, for your own sanity as well as your child's.

When to tell your firstborn about the new baby

Many parents tell their firstborn about their new sibling very early on in the pregnancy, perhaps after the positive pregnancy test or the first scan. Knowing that your child struggles with abstract and hypothetical thinking, a more helpful time to tell them might be closer to the end of your pregnancy. I didn't tell my own children until I was six months pregnant with their future siblings. By this time, we had made any physical preparations necessary (and because they hadn't been told about the new baby's arrival, they didn't link any changes to the baby) and we could really focus on helping them emotionally. Most importantly, though, three months is a long time for little children – and seven, eight or nine months can feel like an eternity. Telling them closer to the baby's arrival meant it was still an exciting idea and they didn't have so long to wait. If you have a very small age gap, you may decide to not tell your firstborn at all.

How to tell your firstborn about the new baby

I don't think there is a right or wrong way to do this. The best way is the one that feels right for you and your child. Some parents plan reveal parties; others just have a very matter-of-fact conversation. Some buy 'new big brother' or 'new big sister' gifts; others use a book to help them explain. The only point that really matters is that when you tell your firstborn, you reassure them that you love them and that that will never change. They need to understand that they are not being replaced or pushed out of your affection. Don't call them 'my big boy' or 'my big girl' – they may feel that being big isn't such a great thing because it means being replaced by somebody little. (This is an idea I'll discuss more in later chapters.) Be ready to answer any questions (especially the 'How-did-the-baby-get-there?' and 'How-will-it-get-out?' ones). Answer them honestly and openly and set their mind at rest as much as you can. Fact is always better than fiction with sex education and birth in particular, however old your child is.

Helping your firstborn to understand what to expect

If your child is slightly older, they are likely to have a much better grasp of what is about to happen, especially if their friends have recently welcomed a new baby to the family. If so, then talking about the new baby, or even visiting the family is a great idea. It really helps to see other children who are new big brothers or sisters, because the tangibility aids abstract thinking. If you don't have any friends or family members with babies, then simply pointing them out when you are out shopping can help. If the babies cry or are being fed, this can spark a conversation about why babies cry (and quite how much) and what they may need. If your child is independently reading, then there are a few good 'big sibling' books on the market (see Resources, page 268). Otherwise, share books together, both non-fiction and fiction.

If your child is younger and not yet able to communicate fully verbally, then share books together (again, see Resources, page 268) and watch programmes with their favourite characters welcoming new babies to their families.

However old your child is, keeping the conversation and exposure going is the best way forward, especially as your due date approaches. The more you talk and share books and films, the more chance there is that it will have a positive effect. Don't rely on just one or two conversations or stories.

Should your firstborn go to scans and appointments?

Involving your firstborn in antenatal check-ups at a clinic or doctor's surgery can be a great way to help them to prepare for the new baby's arrival. However, I'm not a fan of taking a firstborn to scans or hospital appointments for two reasons. The first is that going to a hospital can be a scary experience for a young child – the sounds, the smells, the sight of medical equipment and so on – especially if they have had a traumatic experience at one. The second reason is that medical ultrasounds are not entertainment. Should the sonographer find a problem at your scan, it is probably better if your firstborn is being cared for elsewhere. This also means that you can focus on yourself and the baby, without worrying about how your reactions will affect your firstborn. Standard midwife check-ups, however, are a lovely way to involve your child, especially if the midwife allows them to listen to the baby's heartbeat or explains how the baby is lying in your tummy.

Preparing your child for being left overnight for the first time

Chapter 7 looks in detail at childcare for your firstborn when you're in labour with the new baby. Preparing your child for being away from you while you give birth largely depends on where you will have your baby and how long you will be away from home. (Chapter 6 discusses different options surrounding birthplace.)

For now, if your child is old enough to have a conversation about the new baby, it's a good idea to start dropping little hints about what will happen when the baby arrives, mentioning, for instance, how long you might be away for and who will be taking care of them. As in the case of reducing Mum-centred bedtimes (see page 79), building a strong bond between your child and whoever will care for them while you're in labour is probably the most important thing that you can do. Concentrating on how the caregiver will get your firstborn to sleep comes a close second.

Some other important things mums worry about in advance

Introducing the new siblings

Introducing your firstborn to your new baby is very exciting. Watching two little people that you made meet for the very first time can be emotional for everybody involved. For the smoothest and gentlest introduction, there are a few points that you may want to think about:

- Don't hold your baby when you introduce your first-born to them. Ideally, your baby should be lying in a crib, hospital cot or basket. Having been separated from you for a while, your firstborn is very likely to need a hug and want your arms all to him or herself. Seeing you, or your partner, holding the baby almost lengthens the separation and can cause upset, grief, anger and resentment.

- Introduce the baby as 'our baby' or 'your baby sister/brother'. This gives your firstborn as sense of ownership, which can help to reduce any rivalry.

- Try to cover any blood, bruises or medical equipment, so that your firstborn is not scared when they see you or the baby.

- If you are exhausted or very sore after the birth, it's better to wait a little longer to allow yourself to catch up on sleep, so that you can be enthusiastic and fully welcoming to your firstborn.

- Don't wake your firstborn from a nap or very early in the morning to meet their new sibling. Also, make sure they've eaten first, so they are neither tired nor hungry when they meet their new sibling.

- Ask your firstborn if they would like to stroke or cuddle their new baby sibling, but don't force it. If they say 'no', then accept their decision. There is plenty of time for cuddles in the future.

- Allow and accept any reaction from your firstborn. If they cry, get sad or angry, that's OK. It's a big and confusing moment for them. Don't get upset if their reaction isn't as wonderful as you had hoped.

- Videos and photos are OK, but only if somebody else is taking them and you are free to focus solely on your firstborn. It's a wonderful moment which you will all love to reminisce on as the years go by, but don't sacrifice giving your firstborn your support and full attention in order to capture it.

I spoke to some mothers about the moment they introduced their children for the first time. Here is what they told me:

We introduced our newborn and our eldest at the hospital, a few hours after delivering. He bought his new little sister a balloon and teddy and my partner had bought him the same 'from her' along with a little gift at home for when we all went home.

I had baby number two at home. My daughter was looked after by our neighbours. I left the new baby at home with dad and walked across the road to pick up my daughter. We had a lovely cuddle and chat for five minutes, then I asked her if she wanted to come and see the new baby. Dad then introduced her to him, so I was free to hold her and take pictures.

I made sure that the baby was in the cot asleep when my son came in, so that he could have my full attention. I needn't have bothered as he was desperate to see his brother straight away.

My eldest was two years and three months old when his little sister was born. He met her when she was one minute old (we had a home birth) and I was holding her still in the pool. He'd known what to expect thanks to the books we'd read with him and he was amazed he had a sister. He asked to hold her later that day and has been gentle and affectionate with each day since.

My daughter first met her baby brother at the hospital. It wasn't our original plan, but they were taking their time releasing me. Her first words were, "Oh, Mummy he's so beautiful, can I hold him?"

Should you give your eldest a present from the newborn?

I can't tell you how many times I am asked this question! And my answer is yes to the present, but no to it being from the new sibling.

When your second baby arrives, you may well receive lots of cards and gifts for him or her (albeit not as many as the first time). This can be hard for your firstborn to cope with and to understand. Why is everybody bringing a gift for the baby and not for them? For this reason, I think it's a wonderful idea to give your firstborn a 'new big brother' or 'new big sister' gift and a card (sometimes the cards are more important, as that's what you'll tend to receive the most of), however I would make it from you and not the new sibling. The idea of a newborn baby buying a present is a little silly and unbelievable. I also don't like the idea of the baby having to buy the firstborn's affection. If the gift comes from you though, it's genuine and real and much more believable. It says, 'You are so wonderful. We love you so much. We wanted to buy you this gift.' And that can be so much more powerful. The other thing I always recommend is that if a visitor comes to your house with a gift or card for your newborn, you either ask them to gift your firstborn a little token or, if you don't feel comfortable enough to do that, you can prepare a little basket of small gifts in advance of the new baby arriving and ask your guest to take one and give it to your firstborn. This means that they will feel seen and noticed and appreciated by any visitor who would otherwise shower attention and presents on their new sibling.

Should you encourage your firstborn to choose a gift to give to the new baby? If you have an older child who expresses an interest in doing so, then of course, it's wonderful to honour their request. Otherwise, I don't think this is necessary, since the baby will receive so many gifts anyway. However, what I do recommend is involving your firstborn in as many new-baby purchases as possible: ask them which colour blanket they think the new baby would prefer; let them choose a comforter toy; and ask their opinion on any clothing purchases. As much as possible, try to respect their choices (which may mean allowing some crazy colour combinations). The more they can help to select items for the baby in advance of the birth, the more of a sense of pride and ownership they will have when the baby arrives.

Let's end this chapter with a story from a mum about preparing her daughter for a new sibling, and how the family coped once the baby came home.

Rachel's story

Throughout the pregnancy, my four-year-old daughter, Isabella, was completely involved. She was even the first person to know I was pregnant. My partner, Mark, was at work and Isabella and I got the test and did it together. I was starting to worry I wouldn't get pregnant at this stage (it had been a fair few months) and at first there were no lines. I cried, and Isabella cuddled me and said, 'Don't worry, Mummy, you will get pregnant'. Then we looked a little closer and saw some faint lines. She shared the excitement the entire time, and she also kept it to herself if I asked her to.

She came to the first scan and she came to some midwife appointments. We talked about the baby constantly and acknowledged what would be tricky when baby arrived (sleep, Mummy and Daddy being tired and sometimes cross because of that, sharing, jealousy). We got some books out from the library about having another baby, such as *Mummy, Mummy, What's in Your Tummy?* and our favourite one ever, *15 Things Not to Do with a Baby*, which she now reads to her baby brother.

The day the baby, Callum, was born we made sure that Isabella was the first person other than Mark to meet and hold him. She also got a present and a card from him and it possibly helped that she actually named him too.

From a practical perspective, we made sure that she had moved into her new bedroom a long time before the baby was born, and that she helped decorate it as well as it being completely her choice when she moved into the room. She wasn't ever kicked out of the nursery room. We also made the decision to ditch the toddler bed and keep the double bed in the spare room that became hers. Mark correctly realised before me that one of us would be spending a lot of time in there with her post baby, as well as it giving us the opportunity for more space and sleep. This has helped so much. At first, I could feed the baby at the same time as lying down with Isabella in bed and she would fall asleep, or Mark could put her to bed and lie next to her. As it stands, we essentially both co-sleep with the children, and we switch it up now a bit. So tonight, for example, I have put her to bed while Mark is downstairs with the baby. He will then come into her bed later tonight. It's a win–win: I get to chill without a baby on my boob for a bit, while he gets some baby bonding; then later, he gets to have more sleep in here than in with me and the baby. Isabella wakes up and isn't alone in her room while we are all in the next-door bed. I understand this is probably not ideal for most families, but it suits us.

I hope that this chapter has reassured you in preparing your firstborn for the arrival of their new baby sibling. While a lack of abstract and hypothetical thinking can undoubtedly make emotional preparation hard and less successful than you may have hoped or believed, you'll have seen that there are still plenty of things you can do in advance of the baby's arrival to ease life after the birth and aid the new sibling bond.

Next, I'll be looking at what to keep, what to buy and what the essentials are for life with two children.

Chapter 5

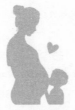

Sorting, Shopping and Sharing

This chapter delves into some of the practicalities of preparing for the transition from one to two children. I'll talk about items that you may want to reuse (and those that you shouldn't), whether sharing items such as toys is a good idea, and how to minimise potential sibling rivalry that may arise as a result of sharing. I'll also look at some of the 'must-have' items for life with two children – with an emphasis on getting out of the house with both of them.

Reusing

One of the big advantages to parenting second time around is that the initial outlay for baby items is dramatically reduced because you can reuse much of what you bought for your first baby. Not only is this a positive for your bank balance, it's also environmentally friendly. The following items are perfect for reusing with your new baby:

- Baby bath and bath seat

- Baby monitor

- Blankets, sheets and sleeping bags

- Changing table and mat

- Clothing

- Cot and crib

- High chair

- Moses basket

- Muslins and reusable baby wipes

- Pushchair and stroller (although you may consider other transport options, discussed later in this chapter)

- Reusable nappies (but be aware that not all nappy types suit all builds; if your babies' body types differ, you may find a different cut will suit them better)

- Slings and carriers (check for any signs of wear that may affect safety, such as fraying)

- Toys (check for signs of wear that may impact safety)

Buying new

Recycling items you used for your firstborn is a great way to save money and help the environment; however, for safety reasons, there are some items that should be buy specifically for your new arrival. These are:

- **Car seats** Car seat recommendations change regularly. For instance, if your first child's second-stage car seat was forward-facing, you may decide to invest in an extended rear-facing seat for your new baby. If the seat is cracked or damaged in any way, the straps are frayed or it has been involved in an accident, then you should buy a new one.

- **Cot and crib mattresses** Research has found that using mattresses previously used by another child can significantly increase the risk of SIDS; however, this effect is most strong if the mattress was previously used by another family.[1]

- **Bottles** Any plastic bottles that are worn or scratched should not be reused, due to the possibility of BPA leakage (a potentially harmful chemical).

- **Bottle teats and dummies** These should always be purchased new for each baby.

- **Nursing bras** Don't assume that you are the same bra size that you were with your first baby – shape and size do change.

- **Anything that may have been recalled for safety reasons since you last used it** Most commonly, recalls occur for toys and safety equipment, such as car seats. You can find a list of current baby product recalls via Trading Standards (see Resources page 269).

New clothes or hand-me-downs

When I had my second baby, I felt torn about reusing clothes from my firstborn. On the one hand, it felt great to recycle and save money. I also loved reusing clothes that had been my favourites with my firstborn; baby clothes get such little wear, it felt fulfilling to give them another outing. On the other hand, something about it made me feel terribly guilty. I couldn't get over the feeling that my second-born deserved to have something new. We had spent hundreds of pounds on new equipment and clothing for our firstborn, I could count on one hand the items we bought new, or new to us, for my second-born. In my more rational moments, I laughed at my anxiety and dismissed it as ridiculous, but in the more emotional ones, the simple act of dressing my new baby in hand-me-downs made me feel so sad for him.

My firstborn was a summer baby and my second-born a winter one. This forced my hand a little, meaning I had to buy some things new for my second son – a snowsuit, for example – but almost everything else was handed down, except for a handful of special outfits. All our newborn-sized clothes tended to be unisex, but even if our first and second babies had been different sexes, I think I would still have reused most of the clothes.

As my second son grew, around 50 per cent of his clothes were handed down from his brother. I also sold a lot of my eldest's clothes, particularly those that were the wrong cut or season. This allowed me to recoup some money, which I spent on buying new, or new-to-us, clothes for my second son. This balance of hand-me-downs and new clothes felt comfortable to me, but there is no right or wrong – just do whatever feels right for you and what you can afford.

To share or not to share?

I am slightly less in favour of passing down toys between siblings. Many parents find that even though their firstborn has outgrown a toy, when they pass it on to their second baby, the firstborn suddenly rediscovers a love for it and is reluctant to share. To get around this, I recommend that you don't pass on toys that were (or are still) precious to your firstborn. If they are old enough to discuss sharing with you, then it's a great idea to go through their toys with them and ask if there are any they would like to pass on to the new baby. If they are reluctant to pass anything on, even if they don't play with it any more, then don't force them. This is a sure-fire way to create problems and sibling rivalry.

I have always tried to make sure that each of my children has their own toys, which are kept in their own spaces (not necessarily their rooms, but in their own toy box or corner of our living room). Those toys remain sacred to each child and they are not forced to share if they don't want to. I think applying this from the very early days is part of the key to its success. This doesn't mean that they never share though; all the bigger purchases, such as garden toys, ride-ons, small-world play and dolls' houses are shared by my children. However, they are shared from the off, and this lack of ownership is important in reducing sibling rivalry in the future.

Essentials with two children

All parents have their own 'must-haves' with two children, but top of a lot of people's lists when they have a second baby is 'a good sling' (I'll talk a little more about this on page 109). The following items are also commonly recommended by parents as essentials:

- Double pushchair
- Buggy board

- Somewhere safe and 'contained' to put the baby down, such as a Moses basket or playpen when they are mobile

- Good breast pump for when you need to be with your firstborn and the baby needs feeding

- Box of toys to keep your firstborn entertained while you feed the baby

- Roomy changing bag to carry the necessities for both children

- Portable changing station, packed in a bag, that you can carry from room to room to avoid leaving the baby and your firstborn alone while you go in search of a new nappy or wipes.

My top tip when purchasing new items for your second baby is to get out any toys or equipment that you buy for them two or three weeks before the due date. This gives your firstborn time to play with them, so that the novelty wears off before the baby is born. If new and exciting toys and equipment suddenly appear once the baby is there, the older child can often struggle with feelings of possessiveness.

Transport options

Depending on the age of your firstborn, it's likely you'll need to consider different transport options for when the new baby arrives. Even if your toddler, preschooler or school-aged child is usually an independent walker and never uses a buggy, it's still best to plan for the days when they will inevitably decide that they are too tired to walk. Here are the main options:

- **Buggy board** This is a good option for an older child to take a ride if they get tired. If they are walking, you can simply hitch the buggy board up out of the way.

- **A sling** This is a 'must-have' with two children. If you buy nothing else, buy a good sling. It means that you can stick with just a regular, single buggy for your firstborn and carry the baby in the sling when you're out and about. At home, the sling allows you to have both hands free for chasing after and playing with your firstborn, while keeping the baby calm. It can be invaluable for bath and bedtimes, too, if you're on your own at night. It means your baby can nap, held securely, without you having to leave your firstborn while you try to get the baby to sleep. And, finally, if you have an inquisitive toddler or preschooler who can't be trusted around their sibling, it also means that the baby is safe when in the sling.

- **Double buggy** Double buggies can be handy if your age gap is small and your firstborn is not quite old enough to ride on a buggy board. They are especially useful if your firstborn still naps (and does so happily in a buggy). The other big – and unintended – benefit I found was that you can sit your firstborn in the buggy, carry your baby in a sling and fill up the other seat with shopping and baby paraphernalia.

Choosing a double buggy

The choice of double buggies on the market seems to grow every year, but how do you know which one is right for you? Here are some points to think about:

- Will you use it immediately or a few months down the line? If immediately, look for one that allows your baby to lay flat, perhaps in a carrycot attachment.

- Does it allow both children to parent-face?

- Will both the baby and your firstborn have a good view? (Some have very restricted visibility for the second child, which can result in tears and tantrums.)

- Does it look comfortable enough size-wise for your firstborn to use for another year?

- How large is it when folded and stored? Will it fit in your car or on public transport easily?

- How long do you think you will use it for? Will it be worth the outlay? What is the resale value?

- Does it convert to a single for when your firstborn has outgrown it?

- How wide is it? Will you struggle to fit it through your front door or shop entrances? (We live in an old market town and many of the shops have very narrow doorways; we quickly discovered that we couldn't fit through about 60 per cent of them when out shopping with our double buggy.)

If you do decide to buy a double buggy, my top tip is to use it with your firstborn for at least a month before the new baby arrives. This means that they will have one less change to deal with the first time you go out with your firstborn and baby in the buggy.

Babywearing

In my experience, babywearing is key to survival in the early days with two children. Using a sling means that you can give your newborn everything they need (namely, physical contact with you) and meet your firstborn's needs too. Having your hands free for your firstborn, whether to play with them, wipe their bottom when they use the potty, make their lunch, dry their tears, give them a bath or tuck them up in bed is invaluable. Slings also make fantastic transport options (we quickly ditched the double buggy and reverted to our regular buggy and a sling). My second-born (and third- and fourth-borns) lived in their slings for their first three months. Nothing we bought was more helpful than the sling when transitioning from one to two children.

The best newborn carriers

If you're new to babywearing, it's crucial to find a sling that works for you. The best way to do this is to find a local baby-wearing consultant or sling library. A quick internet search should direct you to one easily. You will be able to try on different types of slings before you buy and have the bonus of expert advice from experienced babywearers and those who have been on special carrying training courses.

If you can't find a local consultant or group, then the most common sling used for newborns is known as a 'stretchy wrap'. This is a long length of slightly stretchy fabric that initially looks terrifying, but is easy to use once you know how. The illustrations overleaf show how to 'wrap' for a simple newborn hold. Most slings will come with comprehensive instructions and you may find practising with a doll or a teddy bear while watching an online video helpful too.

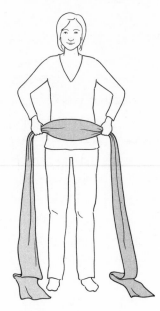

Find the middle of the wrap

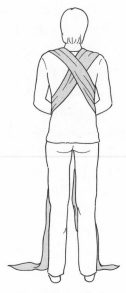

Wrap it around your waist, cross it
behind you and bring the straps up
and over the back of your shoulders

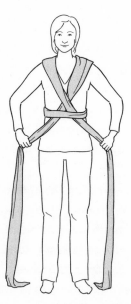

Pass the straps through the band
around your waist and cross them

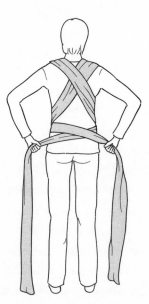

Take the straps around your waist,
cross them behind you and bring
them back to the front

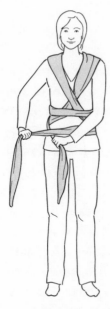

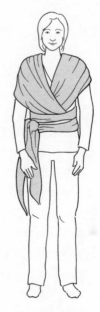

Tie in a double knot at the side.
If there isn't enough fabric to bring
it around to your front, just
tie it at your back

Fan all the fabric out over
your shoulders.

Tandem babywearing

There are ways to carry both children at the same time, usually with the older child on your back and the baby on your front. This requires two different carriers. The older child is often carried in a woven wrap (a thicker fabric with no stretch) or a structured carrier (one with buckles and straps), while the baby is in a stretchy or woven wrap. If you think tandem babywearing is for you, then I would strongly advise you to speak to a babywearing consultant or visit your local sling library.

Carrying in pregnancy

Slings can also be great to use in pregnancy if your firstborn is feeling the need for some extra closeness. There are many ways to carry that don't strain your bump. I happily carried my toddler right up until the very end of pregnancy in a structured carrier on my back. If you are not already an experienced babywearer, then it's definitely a good idea to speak with a babywearing consultant before starting to carry in pregnancy.

Slings can also be a wonderful way to ease any tension in your back and bump during pregnancy. There are certain ways of wrapping them (without a toddler in them) so that they act as a pregnancy support belt, gently holding your muscles and ligaments. This works particularly well at the end of pregnancy when your bump is big. You can also use a shorter woven wrap, or something known as a traditional Mexican rebozo (see Resources, page 269), to help you unwind in pregnancy, get your baby into a good position before the birth and even relax you in labour. This technique is commonly referred to as 'sifting'. You'll find many videos online demonstrating how to do it.

I hope this chapter has helped you to feel a little more prepared for the practicalities of life with two children. Sorting and shopping can be exciting tasks, especially if you share them with your firstborn. Getting all the practicalities sorted – at least mentally, if not in 'real life' – can take a huge weight off your mind and allow you to focus on your pregnancy and the impending arrival of your second baby. This is where the next chapter picks up – planning to give birth for the second time.

Chapter 6

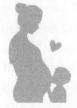

Second Births

How do you feel about giving birth again? Excited? Nervous? Hopeful? Scared? My first birth was a pretty awful experience and I was determined that my second would be different. I realised that if I wanted to make it more positive, it was something that I was going to have research and prepare for myself. But I struggled to find resources. Everything seemed to be focused on birth the first time around. I booked myself into our local NCT refresher antenatal classes, but the emphasis there was much more on coping with two children, than on birthing again. Even the birth books I read seemed to have been written for first-time mothers. I raised my concerns with my midwife at an antenatal appointment and she told me, 'Oh, you'll be fine. You've done it all before, you know what to expect. You're a pro at this now.' But the thing is, I didn't feel like a pro. I felt even more of an amateur than I had first time around. I'd thought I knew what I was doing when I went into labour the first time. I'd thought I was well prepared, but it turned out I wasn't.

Things have moved on since my second baby was born, but

I still feel that the focus in birth preparation and support is on first-timers. In this chapter, I aim to redress this, answering common questions mothers have about giving birth again. I hope to make you to feel more prepared and more reassured and, mostly, to help you to have a positive experience this time, whether you had a great first birth or a difficult or traumatic one.

When I was researching this chapter, I spoke to some mums about their feelings concerning birth the second time around. Here's what they told me:

I'm thirty-four weeks pregnant with number two, and I'm definitely more scared of the birth this time. My first birth (two and a half years ago) wasn't particularly traumatic, but I distinctly remember the pain of the contractions and of the birth itself. People told me you forget the pain, but you don't! However, although I'm more scared, as I know what's to come, I also know I can do it, as I've done it once before. I'll try and keep hold of that thought once my labour starts.

I was so worried about the second birth because the first had some complications – forceps, placenta got stuck, ending up with me being put to sleep for surgery. So I spent a lot of the last weeks worrying. I wish I'd relaxed more because it was a completely different experience – he popped straight out with no worries! Every birth is definitely different.

It may sound silly but I was really worried about giving birth again. Not because my first birth was difficult but precisely the opposite. My first birth was a wonderful experience – better than I had hoped for. I didn't dare hope it would be that easy again. I thought that surely something would go wrong the second time.

I was really excited about my second labour. I couldn't wait to do it all again. My first birth was hard work, but I found it really empowering. That oxytocin high after she was born was amazing. I couldn't wait to experience that again.

I definitely feel more realistic this time. Last time I was all about the candles, the whale music and the meditation. This time I'm more open-minded. We'll see how it goes. I know those things don't really matter. What matters is the people around you. This time my friend is going to be with me, as well as my husband. I think that will really help as my husband was very panicky last time.

Learning from your first birth

If your first birth was difficult or you found it traumatic, the most important and powerful thing you can do is to spend some time finding out what happened – and why. This holds the key for preparing well this time around and reducing any fear and anxiety you may have about doing it again.

Most hospitals offer a 'Birth Afterthoughts' service, where a specially trained midwife will spend some time talking through your notes with you and explaining what happened. This can be invaluable. Similarly, you can request a copy of your notes and go through them. It's helpful if you have a friend who can help with any medical terminology if you don't understand it yourself.

In my experience of teaching antenatal classes to thousands of parents, there are four main elements that build a better experience of birth the second time around:

1. **Understanding** As I've mentioned before, understanding what happened in your labour and birth last time and, most importantly, *why* it happened, is the key to everything else. The power this returns to mothers-to-be can often be immense, especially if they felt powerless the first time around. Understanding also lays the groundwork for the second point: fear-releasing.

2. **Fear-releasing** Giving birth can be a scary and traumatic experience and, sadly, it often is for many. Your birth doesn't have to look stereotypically scary for you to find it traumatic, though. What matters most is how you were treated and how you felt. So even if your birth looked 'perfect' on paper, it is still valid for you to have been scared by it. Similarly, your birth may have sounded traumatic but you may have found it a positive and empowering experience. Any fears that you do retain from your first birth can – and often do – have a strong impact on your second. Releasing these fears is therefore paramount. One way to do this is by gaining an understanding of what happened the first time; the other is by preparing for this time to be different, as covered by the next point.

3. **Preparation** Whether you're a natural planner or you winged your first labour and birth, preparation will play an important role in your labour and birth this time around. For most of you, there will be more to prepare, based on what happened the first time. Whether you are planning a cathartic natural birth, or a calm elective Caesarean, the more you research, plan and prepare before the event, the more chance there is that you will feel in control, calm and confident. Later in this chapter we'll look at the importance of birth plans and why these can look quite different the second time around.

4. **Birth partners** When I worked as an antenatal teacher I discovered that the attitude of the birth partner (whoever they were) to the birth was often a stronger predictor of the outcome than that of the mother-to-be. If the birth partner was nervous, anxious, unsupportive or not particularly interested in learning about birth, the labour was often difficult, as was the birth. There is no coincidence here. Labouring mothers need to feel supported; they need to be surrounded by people who are calm, confident and trusting in her ability to birth. Sadly, all too often this doesn't happen. Spending some time preparing your birth partner and, indeed, carefully selecting them in the first place, can make all the difference this time around. I'll talk about this in more detail a little later in this chapter (see page 132).

Understanding failure to progress

The most common cause of problems and worries that I come across when working with second-time parents-to-be, is that of 'failure to progress' – or longer, drawn-out labours that ended in lots of pain and intervention. Indeed, this is how my own first labour ended. I had planned a home water birth with my first baby. Finally, labour began naturally, just before my forty-third week of pregnancy started. For most of the day, I laboured quietly at home, bouncing on my birth ball, watching television and timing contractions. I was too excited to eat much and definitely too excited to sleep. That evening, I felt things had ramped up a gear and we called the midwife out, who just so happened to be the one that I was hoping for, as she had been present at a home-birth support meeting I had previously attended. I felt in good hands. She examined me and found me to be 4cm dilated. Ecstatic at this news, I jumped into my birthing pool and instantly relaxed. The next few hours went past in a calm, relaxed blur. I napped in between contractions and breathed through them when they came. I remember thinking 'I'm actually really enjoying this!' Then my lovely midwife's shift ended, and she had to go home. Two others replaced her: one qualified and one student. The student was lovely, but I felt uncomfortable with the qualified midwife. She opened the curtains to allow some light from the approaching dawn to come in, as she couldn't see to write her notes. She spoke loudly to the student about me. She asked for my cat (whom I found to be a soothing presence) to be removed from the room and she insisted on getting me out of the pool for regular vaginal examinations because I was 'not dilating quickly enough'. I went from enjoying labour to screaming in pain within an hour of her arrival. The midwife tried to make me have some gas and air, which made me vomit, and kept suggesting that we transfer to hospital for some pain relief as I was clearly not coping. In the moments when she was not in the room, the wonderful student tried to talk me through contractions with breathing and holding my hand. I calmed a little, but it was short-lived. Eventually, I was made to get out of the birthing pool; my temperature had risen a little along with my blood pressure. Because I was 'only seven centimetres', we were persuaded to go into hospital. The twenty-minute ambulance transfer was horrendous. Upon arrival at the hospital, I was diagnosed with 'failure to progress'. They started a Syntocinon drip to speed up my contractions and I begged for an epidural. Thankfully, two hours later my son was born with no other intervention. I found the whole experience extremely traumatic. I felt like a failure: I hadn't tried hard enough to cope with the pain; I wasn't strong enough; I had 'failed to progress'. The words haunted me.

Pregnant with my second baby, I was determined things would be different. I spent hours reading childbirth books and researching clinical studies. I saw a hypnotherapist to help me to reframe the experience in my mind and reduce my fear. I wrote a better birth plan. The more I learned, the more I realised that I hadn't failed at anything. My labour had stalled as a natural response to my discomfort with the second midwife. My body did not feel safe to birth with her around. The lack of support I felt had inhibited my body's release of oxytocin, the hormone of labour, and endorphins, the body's natural painkillers. Everything that happened after her arrival was due to my body responding to the presence of a stressor. I wasn't broken. I knew I could do this again.

Early last century, the British physician Dr Grantly Dick-Read, spoke of what he termed the 'fear-tension-pain cycle', or FTP for short. Dick-Read described the fear of childbirth, based on prevalent negative messages in society and the expectation of difficulty and pain, leading to tension in the body. This tension and anxiety are characterised by an increase in secretion of the stress hormone, cortisol. The body is effectively readying itself to 'fight' or 'take flight' in response to a perceived risk. The secretion of cortisol slows, or halts, labour by inhibiting the body's secretion of oxytocin, the hormone responsible for the progression of labour and stimulating uterine contractions. The increased cortisol also leads to tension and tightness and a lack of oxygenated blood in the uterus, as the fight-or-flight response diverts it to elsewhere within the body, readying it to run away from danger. This reduced blood flow, combined with tightness and tension, leads to pain, causing more fear, more tension and, in turn, more pain, in a never-ending spiral. The further a labouring mother slips into this cycle, the more likely she is to need pharmaceutical pain relief and assistance to birth her baby. The FTP cycle causes long, difficult and painful labour and thus leads to another FTP acronym – 'failure to progress'. The fear-tension-pain cycle was definitely the cause of my 'failure to progress'. Of course, I didn't realise this at the time. I was engulfed in pain, doubt and anxiety. My body was doing exactly what it should do – in response to a perceived threat, shutting down my labour to keep me and my baby safe. When I understood this, I can't tell you what relief I felt, having thought for so long that there was something wrong with my ability to give birth and cope with pain.

Of course, not all 'failure to progress' is caused by the fear-tension-pain cycle. Sometimes there is a physical reason for a tricky labour. Too often, however, the problem is due to women having to labour in conditions that play havoc with birth hormones: being with medical staff who are too 'hands on' (commonly known as 'failure to wait') or not respectful enough of the delicate psychological as well as physiological processes involved in birth; being surrounded by birth supporters who are anxious and share their adrenaline and fear; or being plagued by the subconscious images they take into labour with them (you know the ones you see on television, with women screaming in pain during labour).

Avoiding the fear–tension–pain cycle

The good news is that there are a few simple steps you can take now to reduce the likelihood of slipping into an FTP cycle with your second birth.

- **Regulate your media exposure.** Giving birth always seems to be portrayed as hideously painful and dangerous in fly-on-the-wall maternity-ward programmes, films or sitcoms. And these are the images that lurk in your subconscious, quietly telling your brain to be afraid. Avoid them at all costs!

- **Fill yourself with good birth stories.** People like to listen to a juicy, stressful birth story. In fact, there almost seems to be a taboo around talking about positive ones, with people saying things like, 'There are no medals for doing it without pain relief'. So it's hard to surround yourself with positive birth stories in your everyday life; you must hunt them out, usually in internet discussion groups.

- **Demystify and talk about your previous birth.** See page 117.

- **Pick your birth partners carefully.** See page 132.

- **Think about the environment you will birth in.** In order for the hormone of labour, oxytocin, to flow and help labour to progress well, you need to be in an environment that relaxes you. For some, that is their own home, surrounded by their everyday comforts, which help them to feel calm and rested – much more than they ever could in a hospital or birth centre. Others, however, feel more relaxed in hospital, with the proximity to medical staff and equipment. Think about the lighting too, wherever you are. Bright lights inhibit oxytocin. Battery-operated candles dotted around the room can work well, whether you are at home or in hospital.

- **Consider hypnobirthing, hypnotherapy and mindfulness.** These may sound hippy but all they really involve is getting you into a relaxed state – just as you would be when getting a massage, for example – and helping to reprogramme all the negativity in your mind to something altogether more positive. They also help to teach you relaxation techniques, so that by the time labour arrives, you're a pro (thus avoiding the FTP cycle). There are many different classes you can attend, ideally with your birth partner; or, for a cheaper alternative, investigate books, CDs or online classes.

- **Prepare cues to help relax you before the birth.** When you're in labour, the worst thing you can do is *try* to relax. The harder you try, the more stressed you are likely to feel. (It's a little like trying to go to sleep when you have insomnia.) To avoid the 'trying-to-relax' cycle, which almost always ends in tension, you need to 'condition' some objects to relax you well before labour starts. This could mean, for example, a special blanket that you have curled up with for some time while listening to relaxation recordings, a favourite aromatherapy oil that you diffuse while practising relaxation, or a special piece of music that you have relaxed to many times. When you introduce these cues to the labour environment, your body will have a subconscious relaxation response to them, which means you will relax without having to consciously try.

I utilised all these techniques for my second labour. I had hoped to have a home water birth, but fate had other ideas and I ended up induced a couple of days after my due date because of pre-eclampsia (which hadn't affected me the first time around). The change in location and the absence of water unsettled me a little; however, my relaxation objects, my hypnobirthing practice and the hard work I had done in understanding the FTP cycle gave me flexibility and prepared me well. Ultimately, despite the last-minute change in plans, my second labour was quick, intervention free and an easier, calmer and more positive experience than the first.

FAQs about second births

Here are some of the most common concerns about second births.

I had an instrumental delivery last time – will it happen again?

If your first baby was born with assistance from a ventouse (suction cup) or forceps, the good news is that the risk of this happening again is fairly low at less than 20 per cent.[1] Or, in other words, you have more than an 80 per cent chance of an uncomplicated, spontaneous vaginal delivery this time. Being mindful of the FTP cycle, remaining as active as possible during the first stage of labour, adopting a more upright position in the second stage and avoiding epidural anaesthesia can all help to reduce the risk of needing another instrumental delivery with your second baby.[2]

I had a serious tear last time – does that mean I'll have one this time too?

A third-degree tear involves damage to the perineum and the external anal sphincter muscle. Depending on the severity of the tear, this muscle might be only slightly damaged (a grade 3a tear), moderately (3b) or severely (3c). A fourth-degree tear includes damage to the perineum, external anal sphincter and the interior lining of the bowel, known as the rectal mucosa. Both third- and fourth-degree tears require surgical treatment. Understandably, those who have had serious tears first time around can be very anxious about birthing again. Depending on the severity of the first tear, an elective Caesarean may be offered for the second birth. Alternatively, the chances of a straightforward, serious tear-free, vaginal delivery next time are high, research showing the rate of recurrence at only 1 per cent for those who had a previous third-degree tear and 22 per cent for a previous fourth-degree tear.[3] Given that the risk of recurrence is so low for a third-degree tear, most mothers-to-be will opt for a vaginal delivery with their second baby and, in my experience working as an antenatal teacher and doula, the vast majority don't tear at all second time around. Those who have had a previous fourth-degree tear still have a really good chance of no tearing, or of sustaining a much more minor tear. However, you may want to discuss the idea of an elective Caesarean with your midwife and consultant.

My waters broke before labour last time. Can I help prevent that this time?

Premature rupture of membranes (or PROM) is more likely to occur in a second pregnancy if you experienced it first time around. That said, the risk is still fairly low at 16 per cent.[4] Interestingly, some research has shown that supplementing 100mg of vitamin C daily after the fourteenth week of pregnancy can reduce the risk of PROM for those with a pre-existing history.[5]

Do second babies arrive earlier?

If your first pregnancy felt like it lasted for an eternity, you'll be pleased to hear that second pregnancies tend to be shorter. Research has shown that the average length of a first pregnancy is forty-one weeks and one day, or what we would call 'eight days overdue'.[6] The average length of a second pregnancy, in contrast, is forty weeks and three days, or 'three days overdue'. However, the bad news is that you can expect labour to start only a few days earlier.

Are second labours quicker?

For most first-time mothers, labour is a fairly long process, the average labour and birth lasting for around thirteen hours. The latent phase of labour (the stage at the very beginning of labour, up to 4cm dilatation) tends to last for around six hours, with the active phase of labour (regular contractions, going from 4 to 10cm dilatation) takes another six hours, with an average of 1cm dilatation per hour. Finally, the second stage of labour (where the baby is born) usually lasts for around forty to sixty minutes.

Second time around, the whole of labour and birth tends to be around eight hours long. The latent phase usually lasts for around four to five hours (although lots of false alarms are common in second and subsequent pregnancies). The active phase of the first stage usually lasts for around three hours, with cervical dilatation usually happening at around 2cm per hour. Finally, the second stage of labour tends to last for around twenty minutes for those who have given birth before.

Of course, labour lengths differ hugely from mother to mother and these figures are just a very rough guide.

What if the birth is too quick?

If your first labour was quick, there is a chance that your second may be quicker. This isn't always the case though. And conversely, even if your labour was very long the first time around, there is still a chance that your second labour will be incredibly fast.

I have been present at many second-time births, as a doula, that have taken everybody by surprise. It is not uncommon for me to speak to a second-time mother-to-be about her long and drawn out first labour and then find that everything happens within two hours from start to finish second time around. I've attended six second-time 'born before arrivals' (BBAs) as a doula. Twice, I missed the birth entirely, as did the midwives. After a first labour lasting for the best part of a full day (and night), one mum went to the toilet and very quickly realised she didn't need a poo, as she had thought, but that she was actually delivering her baby. Her husband found her sitting on the bathroom floor with her new daughter in her arms. 'Surprise!' she told him as he entered. Another mum was using the shower to help her through what she thought were early labour contractions. Things quickly ramped up a gear and her baby was born in an undiagnosed breech position, feet first into her husband's arms.

In another case, I supported a mum who was planning a vaginal birth after a Caesarean (VBAC) throughout her second pregnancy. She called me early one evening and told me she thought things were starting. I arrived to find her swaying on a birth ball, eyes closed, listening to her hypnobirthing recording that we had practised together. I asked if she was OK and she smiled and nodded yes. I asked if she felt it was time to go to the hospital and she said, 'No, not yet'. After a quick chat and cup of tea in the kitchen with her husband, I went to check on her again. Not much had changed, except her swaying had sped up and she was now gently humming. Suddenly, she stood up and said, 'The baby is coming!' There was no time to get her to hospital, as originally planned. Dad called the midwives, who called for an ambulance. Mum continued to rock backwards and forwards and caught her baby in her own arms less than ten minutes later, just as the paramedics arrived.

Two more mums I worked with during their second pregnancies had come to me because they had had very long labours – both were diagnosed with 'failure to progress', both needed epidurals and assisted deliveries and experienced a fair amount of birth trauma. The two women had decided to plan home births for their second babies. Both went into labour in the middle of the night, after their firstborns were safely tucked up in bed for the night (a very common occurrence). They laboured calmly and beautifully, trusting their bodies. Within an hour of me arriving, in both cases things changed dramatically and it became obvious they were in the second stage of labour. In both cases, their midwives didn't arrive in time for the birth. The mums got onto all fours and birthed their babies into their own hands. The midwives (and in one case paramedics) arrived to find the new family cuddled up together, happy and smiling. Overwhelmed by how different their experience had been second time around, they both spoke of their 'empowering' second births for years afterwards.

HOW TO COPE WITH A BBA

BBAs (born before arrival) can sound very scary, especially when the news is full of headlines like, 'Hero dad delivers his own baby and saves the day'. Reporters suggest that delivering babies is hugely complex, involving boiling water, lots of towels, dramatic baby 'catching' and the like.

In reality, if the labour is progressing that quickly, the chances are that everything is going perfectly, and when that is the case, nobody really need do anything – the mum does everything herself, instinctively and naturally. There is no need for boiling water, for panic, or for long lists of instructions to follow from emergency-service operators. You simply wait, hold the space, make sure that Mum is comfortable, that the environment is as oxytocin friendly as possible and you allow nature to do its job. You don't need to 'catch' the baby; if Mum doesn't instinctively reach down to it (which, in my experience, all do), then just gently support the baby as it comes out. Be on hand with some dry, fluffy towels (the only thing you do really need) to wrap up Mum and baby together and keep them warm. And pop some towels over any furniture or carpets you would like to protect. Don't worry about dressing the baby (they get all the heat they need from skin-to-skin with Mum) and leave the cord well alone. If you have called the midwife or ambulance, quickly go and open your front door and leave it ajar, so that you can stay with Mum and they can let themselves in. Keep the phone near to you, but try to focus on Mum, rather than constantly talking with the person on the end of the telephone. The most important thing for you to do is to stay calm. Women have been doing this for thousands of years!

Choosing where to give birth

When I taught antenatal classes, I always used to get parents-to-be to draw a picture of their ideal relaxation environment – somewhere that made them feel calm, at peace, comfortable and able to really let go of the 'noise' of the rest of the world. I asked them to think specifically about lighting, sounds, smells, objects that provided comfort and where they would sit. Their pictures often included beaches and oceans, often lit by moonlight; or cosy living rooms with furry throws, open fires, candles, soft music and scents of flowers, vanilla, baking bread or just 'fresh' smells.

After they had drawn their pictures, I asked them to draw their ideal birthing environment, either as the labouring mother or as her partner, supporting her in an environment that felt nurturing and calming. The pictures were almost always identical to the first ones, although fewer were outside in nature, with more in cosy living rooms. However, not one of the thousands I taught ever drew a traditional hospital room.

We discussed why it was that they never drew a hospital – even those who were certain that they wanted a hospital birth. They all agreed that while some felt safer in a hospital, they were generally not as birth-friendly – or, rather, oxytocin-friendly – as other environments they had envisaged. My goal here was to get the parents-to-be to think more about their surroundings and, most importantly, what they could take from their drawings and apply anywhere. So those birthing in hospitals could take a soft blanket from home, aromatherapy oils to spritz in the room, battery-operated candles, some music to listen to and sunglasses (to block out some light and provide privacy).

Many chose to book a home birth after doing this exercise, although this wasn't my intention. It is always possible to make the most of a birthing environment, wherever you are, and the best one for you is the one you feel safest and most comfortable in – for some, that is a hospital or a birth centre; for others, that is at home.

Is home birth a safe and viable option?

In the UK, between 2 and 3 per cent of babies are born at home each year.[7] For first-timers, as happened to me, planned home births often end up in transfers into hospital. Usually, this is not because of an emergency but because of 'failure to progress'. The risk of transfer is significantly lower for second-time births, with most planned second-time home births occurring successfully at home.

Research has shown that planned home births, attended by a midwife, are just as safe as births in hospital, for both baby and mother.[8] Births that are planned to be at home result in fewer Caesareans, assisted deliveries and third- or fourth-degree tears, less postpartum haemorrhage (extremely heavy bleeding) and less need for newborn resuscitatation.

BOOKING A HOME BIRTH 'JUST IN CASE'

When I was teaching antenatal classes, if a family were on the fence about where to have their baby, I always suggested that they speak to their midwives about booking a home birth with the possibility of going into hospital on the day, if that's what they instinctively felt was best once labour started. This is the only way to keep options open, allowing you to make the decision at the last minute. (You can't book a hospital birth and decide on the day that you'd rather stay at home.) The other benefit of this 'hedging-your-bets' approach is that should labour happen quicker than you expect, everything is in place for a last-minute home birth.

Choosing your support team

I've already looked at the role of birth partners a little in this chapter, but as their attitude and approach can and will have a huge impact on your labour it's something I'd like to return to. If your birth partner is scared, nervous or even reluctant to be there, you will pick up on their concerns and there is a strong chance that this will send you spiralling into the FTP cycle (see page 121).

For the easiest, smoothest experience, you want a birth partner who is confident in the process of birth, believes that you can do it, stays calm and supports you and makes sure that your birth wishes are adhered to as much as possible. In a sense, they need to incorporate the role of bouncer, butler and meditation coach! I have worked with some amazing partners, who filled all these criteria and then some. I've also worked with some who needed extra support on the day. That support can take the form of a family member or close friend who you trust to support your wishes and, ideally, who has had great experiences of childbirth themselves. Using a birth partner who themselves had traumatic births or who hasn't yet given birth or witnessed it can mean added anxiety in the birthing room, which is something you really don't need. This is where a doula comes in.

A doula will work to support the mum and her partner, not just during the labour and birth, but in the run-up too. They provide practical care (I have filled many birthing pools, made endless cups of tea and held many sick bowls) and emotional support (lots of reassurance – for both parents – talking through breathing techniques and encouraging smiles) and can also help to decipher medical speak and make sure your birth preferences are followed as closely as possible. Sadly, they are not free. You can expect to pay £500–2000, depending where you live and on how experienced the doula is (whether they are fully qualified or still in training). Many doulas accept payment plans and there is also a special access fund that helps to provide doula support for those on a low income (see Resources, page 269, for more details).

Writing a birth plan

The beauty of a birth plan lies not necessarily in the plan itself, but in the time taken to research, think about and discuss your wishes and hopes with your birth partner/s. Making sure your birth partner knows what is on your birth plan and understands it all is so important. Too many mothers-to-be write birth plans for their baby without any input from the birth partner. They need to be written and discussed together well in advance of the birth.

So how do you write a great birth plan?

- **Keep it short.** Ideally, it should be no longer than one side of A4 paper.

- **Use bullet points.** This makes it easier to read, rather than long sentences and paragraphs.

- **Keep it flexible.** I always prefer to call them 'birth preferences', rather than 'birth plans'. Giving birth can – and does – take unexpected turns, so being flexible with this, rather than having a rigid plan, is so important. Think about all eventualities. For instance, if you're planning a home birth, include a section about what would happen if you were in hospital. Or, if you're planning a VBAC (vaginal birth after a Caesarean), write a section about what you'd like to happen if you do end up with a repeat Caesarean.

- **Think about what matters to you the most.** Don't feel the need to fill the plan up with points that are not so important to you just because those sections appear on sample birth plans you've come across in magazines or on the internet.

- **Include a section for your birth partner to follow.** For instance, you might want to give them instructions for setting up your birth environment once labour starts.

- **Print several copies.** You'll need one for your birth partner to keep as a memory jogger on the day and some for any medical professionals you meet in labour. They have a habit of going missing!

It's never too early to begin writing a birth plan – the earlier you start, the more you can research and understand your options. Ideally, however, you would want to have written your plan by around thirty-six weeks of pregnancy, although even after this you can continue to tweak it – right up until the day your baby arrives.

When writing this book, I spoke with several mums about their births the second time around, after previously traumatic or difficult first labours and births. Debbie and Anna were two of them. What I love about their stories are the themes of knowledge, support and empowerment that suffuse their second births. A positive experience is not about having a 'perfect' drug-free natural birth; it's about having the birth that is right for you and your baby – one where you feel supported and respected, just as Debbie and Anna did.

Debbie's story

I had a traumatic birth with my first: a long labour, back-to-back position, stuck at 9.5cm dilated for hours and with a maximum dose of Syntocinon to try to speed things up. I was exhausted. I ended up with an epidural, followed by a failed attempt to deliver via ventouse and then forceps and a third-degree tear. My doctor had sweat on her upper lip trying to get the baby out. I had to be stitched in the operating theatre, while my newborn was left with Dad. The stitches resulted in painful walking and sitting for a long time after his birth, something I hadn't anticipated or been prepared for. I also had an altered physiology in my perineum following the stitches. I was worried that this or worse (a greater tear) would happen again and cause more long-term damage. My midwife, however, thought it wouldn't, as I was much more active during my second pregnancy – I had a toddler and spent lots of time pretending to be a dog or a dinosaur! I also worked until later on in the pregnancy, but I still had an extra appointment with the hospital midwife to put in place a more detailed birth plan.

In the end, I went into labour naturally at midnight on my due date. Contractions were five to six minutes apart throughout. I stayed at home as long as possible, for my toddler's sake, though we had to phone a friend at two o'clock in the morning for them to come and take him to their house. By this time, I was having almost constant contractions. On arrival at the labour ward, I was sent to the waiting room, but didn't make it. On examination I was already 10cm dilated and, after only three pushes, my daughter was born. It was a shock that the birth was so fast and easy, and so different. This time it was only three and a half hours, compared to twenty hours of exhaustion. I could feel it – feel her being born, which was amazing to me, as I'd had an epidural with my firstborn. And I'm so thankful for that. Plus, I had only one tiny little tear second time around.

Anna's story

My first experience of motherhood was not as I'd expected . . . I feared the birth part (I think that's quite normal), but it was still a shock when things started to go wrong. My waters broke in the early hours and the contractions started immediately at ninety seconds apart. Excited that it was all kicking off, my husband rang the hospital and I eagerly followed their advice and went in straight away. I was monitored and found out that baby's heart wasn't really liking the contractions. I had an examination and discovered I was only 2cm dilated. Because of the intensity of the contractions they wouldn't send me home again, but I also couldn't be admitted. So there I was, in limbo. I was put in a side room and somewhat forgotten. I kept sending my husband out and he was told, 'We'll be with you in a minute'. I wasn't allowed any gas and air, because I hadn't been admitted, so I just remained in limbo for what felt like an eternity. I was confused. I didn't understand at the time that I hadn't been admitted properly and got upset and frustrated at not receiving the attention I felt I needed. When I was finally admitted, I was told they needed to test the oxygen levels in the baby's blood. They took a sample from her head, but the equipment got stuck, so it remained in her head and I was told they would remove it once she was born. I wanted an epidural. The first one didn't work, the second had to be re-sited and the third one, thankfully, took hold. After thirty minutes of respite, I was then told I needed an emergency section after thirty-six hours of labour. The equipment in baby's head needed removing – so in she went, up to the elbow!

In the operating theatre, I could feel what was going on and had a little freak-out (I later learned it was a normal sensation). The anaesthetist turned to me and said, 'If you can't cope with this I'm going to have to put you out' – and just like that, without any discussion, I was put under general anaesthetic and missed the birth of my baby girl. When I came round, I was groggy and disoriented. By this time, it was late. I got moved onto the ward and my husband was told to leave. I was alone, confused and responsible for this new little baby that I could hardly even hold.

By Day 5, my daughter's weight had dropped too low as she was not getting enough from me breastfeeding (I always blamed her traumatic arrival for my lack of milk, but I've since discovered I just don't really make any). I'd never been sure if I wanted to breastfeed until I couldn't, and then it was then the only thing in the world I wanted. We were readmitted to hospital to get her weight up. After she put on weight overnight, we were discharged and ready to start our journey as a family of three. It wasn't easy. I felt robbed. Robbed of my birth, robbed of the first cuddle, robbed of that precious bonding time when I couldn't hold her because I was having a transfusion or intravenous antibiotics, robbed of breastfeeding and robbed of half of my husband's paternity leave. It took six months before I started to recover, stopped crying every single day and started to focus on building a bond with my baby. I had counselling, my relationship with my husband suffered and we tag-teamed on who was struggling most.

Two years later, we made the decision to have another baby. I was adamant that I was not going to have a repeat experience. I wanted a home birth; I didn't want to set foot in a hospital again. My community midwife was incredible. She spent hours with me at my house, helping me with my birth plan. She arranged for me to have meetings with senior staff at the hospital to talk through my plans, how I felt last time and what they could do to help me feel comfortable this time around. Reluctantly, I was convinced to have my baby in hospital on the condition that I would stay at home for as long as possible (I was convinced – and still am – that half of the problem was that I wasn't free to move around in labour), would go to the low-risk rooms and if I needed to be more closely monitored at any point, things would constantly be evaluated and I would go back to low risk as soon as possible.

The day arrived. I woke at two o'clock in the morning, to the unmistakable squeeze of labour. Up we got, the candles were lit, the classical music played, the doula arrived and my parents were called to come and look after my daughter. At just before seven o'clock, we left for the hospital when I couldn't really handle the pain any more and needed more than paracetamol and my TENS machine. It was a car journey I don't ever wish to repeat, but we arrived. My waters broke in the car in the car park. I hobbled across the tarmac and eventually made it into the birthing suite. I got on the gas and air and was examined and told I was ready to go. Two pushes later and she was out and placed into my arms.

From the horrendous experience of my first birth, I had just managed a six-hour unmedicated VBAC. I was so incredibly proud of myself. The bond was instant. I still struggled with breastfeeding but I handled it a lot better this time. I'm now a confident mum of two and love spending time with them both. I'm so proud of what I achieved – so much so, I want to do it again!

Birth after a previous Caesarean section

If your firstborn was born via a C-section, depending on the reason for delivery, you may be able to choose between a vaginal birth after C-section (VBAC) or an elective repeat C-section (ERCS) with your second baby. Making the decision to have a

VBAC or an ERCS is an easy and straightforward one for many second-timers. Some know what they want to do with certainty as soon as they find out they are pregnant again, or even before; for some, the decision is harder; and for others, the decision is a purely medical one and out of their control.

If you have the option to decide, but are struggling to reach a decision, the table below covers some of the most common reasons why people choose to have a VBAC or an ERCS.

VBAC	ERCS
To take back control and heal after a previously traumatic birth experience.	To avoid going through another traumatic birth experience.
To reduce the risks posed by another C-section (such as infection).	To reduce the risks posed by a natural birth (perineal trauma, for instance).
To reduce the amount of time spent in hospital, away from your firstborn.	To reduce the uncertainty surrounding the birth, allowing you to plan and prepare your firstborn for your absence.
To speed up postnatal healing, so you can get back to normal as quickly as possible to take care of your two children.	To avoid a potential emergency C-section which may lead to longer healing time.
Because you may be thinking of having more children and want to avoid another C-section to reduce risks for future pregnancies.	Because there are questions surrounding your chances of a successful VBAC, such as having placenta praevia in your second pregnancy, large fibroids, a breech presentation or a bicornuate (heart-shaped) uterus. (Note: these do not necessarily preclude a successful VBAC).

Choosing a VBAC

If your pregnancy is an uncomplicated singleton pregnancy (one foetus), with a cephalic (head-down) baby that goes full term (i.e. labour doesn't start before thirty-seven weeks), then your chance of a successful VBAC is around 75 per cent.[9] These are good odds, but you can push them even more in your favour by following as many of the points in the list below as possible:

- Understand the reason for your C-section with your first baby, especially any role that FTP may have played.

- Release as much fear and anxiety surrounding your first birth as you can. Learn hypnobirthing or meditation techniques to help you to relax.

- Surround yourself with positive VBAC stories – join a VBAC support group, either in 'real-life' or via an internet forum.

- Consider your birthing place carefully. Where will you feel safest and most relaxed?

- If you plan a hospital birth, make sure you meet your the consultant midwife to discuss your VBAC options in advance and ask for any agreements to be written down, so that your birth partners can share the evidence on the day.

- Choose your birth partners well. Who will help you to feel confident and calm? Consider employing a doula who is experienced in VBAC births.

- Stay active and healthy throughout your pregnancy. Try to limit weight gain. Practise exercises to help your baby get into the best position for birth (see Resources, page 269).

- Consider seeing an osteopath or chiropractor if your baby got 'stuck' in your first labour, to help your pelvis accommodate your baby in the best position.

- Write a great birth plan and make sure your birth partners understand it fully before labour begins and uphold as much of it as possible when it does.

- Try to avoid unnecessary practices during labour, which can lead to over-medicalisation of the birth process and what is known as the 'cascade of intervention'. For instance, vaginal examinations and continuous monitoring do not significantly improve outcomes, but can lead to more intervention.

- Allow labour to begin naturally when your body and baby are ready.

- Stay active during labour; move around as freely as possible. Get up off the bed and rock on a birthing ball or stand and circle your hips. Rest in a kneeling-on-all-fours position rather than lying on your back.

- Avoid lying on your back during the second stage of labour in order to make optimum space in your pelvis for the baby to be born.

- Believe in yourself. You can do this!

Risk of scar rupture

One of the top worries surrounding a VBAC is that of scar rupture (the previous C-section scar breaking down). Scar rupture is potentially a very serious event that requires immediate surgical intervention. It is, however, very, very rare affecting only 5 out of every 1000 women who have had a previous C-section. This translates to around a 0.5 per cent risk, which may increase slightly in women who get pregnant quickly after their first baby (a gap of twelve months or less between births), are obese, have a baby weighing over 4.5kg (10 pounds), are over forty years old, have a pregnancy lasting beyond forty weeks or show thinning of the lower segment of their uterus on an ultrasound.[10]. But even with these risk factors, the risk is still low.

Frequently asked questions about VBAC

Choosing a VBAC can raise many questions; here are the most common that mothers tend to ask.

When do you have to decide by?

When you find out that you are expecting your second baby, it is understandable that your thoughts turn quickly to giving birth. You may be asked about your hopes for your birth when you first meet with your midwife, but you really don't need to make any decisions early on. The general consensus is that you should do so by the time you are thirty-six weeks pregnant, giving you – and the medical staff caring for you – time to prepare for your baby's arrival.[11] Of course, the earlier you decide, the more time you will have to prepare, but don't feel pressured into deciding in the first – or even the second – trimester of your pregnancy.

What if you had placenta praevia with your first baby?

One of the reasons you may have required a C-section for your first baby is placenta praevia, where the placenta grows very close to or over the opening of the cervix, making a vaginal birth either dangerous or impossible. Research shows that there is a 1 per cent increase in the risk of a placenta praevia with a second pregnancy if you had it first time round.[12] In other words, the chances of needing another C-Section for the same reason is very, very small.

Can labour be induced with a VBAC?

Inducing labour after a previous C-section is a controversial topic. Many hospitals prefer to avoid induction using artificial oxytocin drips or prostaglandin (hormone) pessaries, but will consider an artificial rupture of membranes (breaking your waters). Unfortunately, the evidence showing the safety of induction for VBACs is not conclusive[13], so decisions tend to happen very much at an individual level, depending on the pregnancy and the policies of the hospital.

In fact, for the best chance of a successful VBAC, labour should, ideally, start naturally, meaning that your baby and body are optimally ready for birth.

Does a VBAC have to mean being constantly monitored?

Current guidelines suggest that women who have a VBAC should be offered continuous electronic foetal monitoring (CEFM). CEFM is used to monitor the baby's heart rate and the strength of contractions throughout labour, via electronic pads fixed to the mother's stomach, usually with an elasticated belt. Some hospitals have wireless machines, allowing the mother some freedom of movement; others require that she stays fairly still because of the wires attaching the pads to the monitor.

The idea behind CEFM is to keep a closer eye on the progress of labour and the baby's reactions, which allows medical staff to spot any problems. However, while the machine may constantly monitor, unless a midwife or doctor is continuously monitoring the output, it is arguably no better at picking up problems than intermittent listening with a sonicaid (the portable device midwives use to listen to the baby's heartbeat during antenatal appointments), as found in a recent review.[14] Similarly, CEFM does not reduce the number of baby deaths. It does, however, increase the number of C-sections performed and thus reduces the likelihood of a successful VBAC. For this reason, many VBAC mothers refuse CEFM and instead opt for intermittent monitoring with a hand-held sonicaid.

Is a VBAC possible at home (HBAC)?

Research has found that women who plan to have their VBAC at home have a significantly higher chance of achieving a successful one, compared to those birthing in hospital.[15] The same research has found that statistically, there is no higher chance of complications or adverse outcomes for either mothers or babies with VBAC home births compared to hospital VBACs. There is, however, a fairly high transfer rate, with a third of planned home VBACs moving to hospital, although this may be due to maternal request or attending midwives being slightly more nervous attending a home VBAC, compared to a non-VBAC home birth. So this transfer rate could potentially be reduced with good emotional preparation and by being surrounded with confident birth partners and caregivers.

A better question to ask, perhaps, would be 'Why plan a home VBAC?' The answers here are overwhelmingly to escape hospital policies which may interfere with the likelihood of a successful VBAC, to be able to use a birthing pool, to be surrounded by midwives you probably know and to be in an environment where you already feel safe and relaxed. Of course, this only applies if you believe that you would feel safer at home than in hospital.

Is a water birth possible with a VBAC?

Although, at the time of writing, there is no study looking at the safety of water birth relating specifically to VBACs, research shows that it does not put babies, or labouring mothers, at any extra risk, compared to labour and birth on 'dry land'.[16] Mothers who labour and birth in water report lowered pain and anxiety levels and need less pain relief and medication to speed up labour. Water birth, therefore, seems the perfect accompaniment to a VBAC. The difficulty, however, lies in a hospital VBAC, both in avoiding continuous electrical monitoring and being allowed to use the hospital birth pool, when you are considered higher risk. For this reason, many women who hope to labour and/or birth in water for their VBAC plan to birth at home, where they can avoid constant monitoring and use their own hired or cheaply bought inflatable birth pool.

I spoke to some mothers who planned a VBAC for their second babies. Here are two of their stories:

Jo's story

My first child was breech and born by planned Caesarean section. It wasn't the birth I had hoped for, so second time around I was excited at the prospect of experiencing contractions and going into labour. Being a VBAC, the hospital wanted me to birth on the labour ward, something I didn't want to do unless medically necessary. So we liaised with the consultant midwife and she worked with us to prepare a birth plan to have our baby on the midwife suite. After much research, we decided that it was our preference to have a home birth. At the very least, I wanted to give myself what I felt to be the best opportunity to labour at home for as long as possible. It was quite late on in my pregnancy (around thirty-four weeks) and it involved registering with the home-birth team at another hospital. And although the aim was to have a home birth, since it would be a VBAC we were fully prepared for the possibility of having the baby at hospital. I was feeling very positive about the birth and that we had every possibility available to us. I felt empowered and excited.

On the day I went into labour, I experienced cramps all day, but thought nothing of it because we had had a previous false alarm a few days earlier. As the evening wore on, my cramps intensified and it became clear they were not just cramps but contractions. Our doula came over around 10pm. We laughed and joked, and she suggested we all go to bed and get some rest. Once I went to the dark and quiet of my bedroom the contractions suddenly ramped up a lot. I was now unable to function normally between them. Our doula returned around midnight. I was on the couch and she sat on the floor beside me and spoke softly and calmly. She told my husband to call the midwives and asked me to get into a position to try and slow the labour to give the midwives time to arrive. But suddenly I felt the urge to bear down. I got on the floor, leaned over our footstool and said I needed to push. My doula told me to do whatever felt instinctive. I felt completely calm and in control. I just went with it. I didn't think about the fact the midwives hadn't arrived yet! The thought didn't even cross my mind.

Just as my doula was helping take off my pyjamas, a big contraction came. I pushed hard and suddenly my baby was born! I picked her up and felt a huge surge of love and ecstasy. We sat there like that, looking at one another. It was perfect. It was quiet, intimate, undisrupted. The midwives arrived around 15 minutes later.

Quite astonishingly, my toddler, who was upstairs, had slept through everything and slept until late that morning. So I was able to just sit in the comfort of my own home, on my own couch, with my dog, a cup of tea and my beautiful new baby to enjoy.

Susie's story

Both my husband and I were desperate not to have another C-section with our second baby. We'd both had a stressful experience with our first baby's birth, even though the C-section was planned and everything from a medical perspective was uncomplicated. Emotionally, we found the hospital experience distressing and my recovery was more painful and longer than we both had anticipated. By comparison, the feelings I experienced with my VBAC were immense. The oxytocin high seemed to last for weeks. I felt physically and emotionally strong, not weak like I had after my section. My husband was free to drink up all the joy, not worried and anxious about my wellbeing as he had been after the section.

My top tips for others considering a VBAC are to iden-tify what your concerns with having one might be and address them. If you like being informed, then read. Lots. Talk to the consultant midwife at your hospital's midwife suite. She is the most experienced midwife and the one who can talk you through all your options. Guidelines are just that. They are not written in stone and it is your choice how you labour. The consultant midwife will work with you to write a birth plan for the other health professionals to follow. You can decide, within reason, how many vaginal examinations you have, type of monitoring, communication and so on. I'd also suggest you talk to the lead midwife of the home-birth team. They tend to be very woman-focused and will be happy to chat, regardless of whether you decide to have a home birth. Hire a doula if your budget allows – one with VBAC experience. They will help you navigate the hospital hurdles and help make sure the setting and environment are as conducive to a VBAC as possible. They can be a terrific source of experience, providing guidance and support throughout your pregnancy and birth.

Until I had my VBAC I didn't think I needed any emotional healing following the section. I'm just not that kind of person. I'm a practical, tell-it-how-it-is kind of person. But in the weeks following my VBAC, I realised the whole experience had been incredibly healing. I had successfully laboured. I felt every contraction, the waters break, delivered a placenta, held my baby skin-to-skin the moment she arrived. I was successfully breastfeeding. The emotional healing I experienced changed me for ever. The physical healing following my VBAC was incredibly quick and easy. My uterus contracted quickly, my bleeding was minimal, I felt strong, almost energised. I had second-degree tearing, which healed quickly and without issue and, most importantly, I was quickly able to run around after my toddler!

Planning an elective Caesarean section

If you don't feel that a VBAC is for you, or if you know that your second baby will need to be born via an elective C-Section, there are many things you can do to make the experience a positive one. When speaking to mothers who had had two C-sections, I found that there was one overwhelming message coming through – that of control. I don't think you can over-estimate how important feeling a sense of control over your birthing experience can be. The more in control you feel, the more empowered you will be. This is one place where elective C-sections differ so much from the emergency ones that many go through the first time around. With an emergency C-section, it can often feel as if events are happening to you, and you have very little say, nor any ability to change them. With an elective C-section, you very much have a say and can plan the birth day well in advance. The result is usually a much calmer, far more positive experience that usually results in quicker postnatal healing, both physically and emotionally.

Here's what some mothers told me about their experience of elective C-sections:

I had to have an elective Caesarean (as I had had an emergency one the first time). I was really nervous about it beforehand, but the midwife and anaesthetist worked really hard to calm me down and it was much better than I expected.

My first child was born via emergency C-section. My obstetrician recommended an elective section when I was pregnant with my second child, to avoid the risk of the same problem potentially occurring (placental abruption). I felt comfortable with his recommendation, and knowing the date upon which my son would arrive made it easier to arrange care for my daughter who was only eleven months old at the time. I knew what to expect after the emergency section previously, but it was a much calmer experience and I could take more of it in, rather than stressing as I did the first time. As it was planned and not rushed, my recovery was much quicker, and it was less painful, I found. I also knew what clothes to pack to make dressing easier and more comfortable, etc. My husband could also plan leave from work and found it easier not seeing his wife in pain during labour.

I planned an elective section with my second baby. It was an amazing experience compared to the emergency one I had first time. It was so calm and enjoyable. I'm so pleased I didn't try for a VBAC.

The 'natural Caesarean'

In recent years, the idea of the 'natural Caesarean' has gathered increasing interest and support. [17] The idea behind it is to mimic a natural vaginal birth as much as possible. The baby is delivered slowly, sometimes 'crawling' out of the uterus themselves, providing a much calmer and less stressful experience for the baby. The umbilical cord is allowed to pulsate before being cut, meaning that the baby's blood inside the cord drains back into their body, rather than being lost to them with premature cutting of the cord. Lights are often dimmed, screens are dropped to allow parents to see their baby being born and skin-to-skin contact happens in the operating theatre, providing a head start to bonding and the initiation of breastfeeding. This process is not only beneficial to babies, but to the new parents too, who find the whole process nurturing and beautiful in a way that isn't usually associated with what is essentially major surgery. The parents, rather than being passive bystanders, play an active role in their baby's birth.

While it is rare to find a hospital offering a full natural C-section experience, many will entertain at least some of the features, such as dropping the screens for parents to witness the moment of birth, immediate skin-to-skin contact and delayed cord clamping, if all is well with the baby.

Writing a birth plan for an elective Caesarean

Many parents seem to think that birth plans are only appropriate for vaginal births. This could not be further from the truth. Birth plans are just as important for C-sections, if not more so. Writing the plan allows you to research different options available to you and helps you to feel as in control of the experience as possible. As before, you should discuss your birth plan with your birth partner and make sure that they fully understand your wishes. Print several copies and ask any medical staff involved in your care at the hospital to read over it, preferably in advance of your baby's birth day, but at least as soon as you meet them on the day.

Here are some points to consider when writing a C-section birth plan:

- If you have an option regarding appointment time, aim for a slot as early in the day as possible. This means there will be less chance of you being 'bumped' later in the day, or even to the next day, should emergencies arise.

- Would you prefer to opt for a catheter or not? Not having one can reduce the chance of discomfort and infection. It just means that you will have to go to the toilet as much as possible beforehand and get up and about earlier after.

- Do you want to go to the operating theatre in a wheelchair or to walk down yourself (either is fine, even though most opt to be wheeled down)?

- Would you like the staff in the operating room to chat with you to put you at ease? Or would you rather they were as quiet as possible, perhaps to allow you to focus on meditation or relaxation techniques.

- Will you want to play your own music in the theatre? (And if so, make sure you have it to hand on the day.)

- Might you want to use your own towel and blanket in theatre for your baby, rather than the rather scratchy hospital ones?

- Ask when your birth partner can take photos in theatre, and whether any video is allowed.

- If you don't know what sex your baby is, would you prefer that you and your partner be allowed to discover for yourselves, rather than staff announcing, 'It's a boy!' or 'It's a girl!'?

- Consider asking for the baby to not be wiped or cleaned at all, to allow the vernix to absorb (this is better for their skin).

- Raise the possibility of delayed cord clamping to allow the baby's blood (in the umbilical cord) to return to their body.

- Ask whether the screen can be lowered while your baby is delivered, so you can watch him or her being born (it will be put back in place before you are stitched up).

- Ask if your partner can stay (with you and the baby) while you are stitched up. If they are not allowed to stay, decide whether you want the baby to stay with you, or wait in recovery with your partner.

- Will you be given an opportunity for skin-to-skin contact in the theatre? And if you are unable to hold the baby yourself, can somebody hold them skin-to-skin to you?

- If you are planning to breastfeed, ask for help in lifting your baby to you during your stay, if no co-sleeper crib is provided and if you are too stiff or sore to lift them unaided.

- Ask for peppermint tea after the operation (it's best to take your own with you) to try to allay some of the famous post C-section wind.

Megan's story is a wonderful example of how positive an elective C-section can be, especially if your first birth was by an emergency one:

Megan's story

My first birth was not what I had expected. I had prepared for an active birth. Unbeknown to anyone, I had a constriction band on my uterus, so there was no way my baby was coming vaginally. After a long labour and failed assisted birth they did an emergency C-section and found I'd also ruptured my uterus. I was drained physically and mentally and felt I was a failure. I didn't even know my baby had been birthed until I saw him from a distance and they cleaned him, wrapped him up and took him off to weigh him. My memory was hazy, and I couldn't picture my newborn baby being born. Where was my natural, messy baby skin-to-skin? We were incorrectly told not to take photos, so I didn't have a first photo for hours. This all led to me struggling with post-birth traumatic stress and I was referred to a consultant psychologist who helped me reconstruct my memory and emotionally heal.

When I fell pregnant again, I already knew I had to have a planned C-section. They didn't want to risk me having any contractions, so I was booked in for 39 weeks. I did a lot of research about C-sections – it's not something they cover in antenatal classes. I knew I wanted and needed a positive experience this time. So I decided I would try hypnobirthing and have a natural C-section, also known as a woman-centred C-section. The hypnobirthing would require me to have my music playing in theatre. The natural section meant I didn't want a drape, so I could watch the birth. I wanted the birth to be slow and allow my baby to birth himself with as little assistance as possible from the surgeon. Among other specifics, I wanted to watch the cord pulsate and drain, have immediate skin-to-skin in an untouched state, no unnecessary checks until later, microbiome seeding and to be left alone to allow breastfeeding to be initiated with a breast crawl. I took control and wrote a very detailed birth plan and arranged a meeting with the supervisor of midwives and surgeon to ensure my wishes could be met. The team were fantastic, accommodating and willing to try new things and support me. This included my insistence that I bedshare with my baby during my time in hospital. (Following my first C-section my baby was in the hospital crib and I was unable to move to get him when he cried for milk.)

When the day arrived, it was such a different experience! Exciting and calm. It all went to plan and was a totally amazing event; I can remember so vividly watching him take his first breaths and being placed straight on my chest. The midwife captured some beautiful photos of the whole birth and my husband was at my side. He cut the cord and I held my baby skin-to-skin the whole time I was being stitched up and through to recovery where he did a breast crawl. I really would have loved to have a VBAC, but I can honestly say this experience was amazing and positive. The recovery was so quick; I went home the next day! The key thing is to be positive and take control. Do your research and find out what you can ask for. Meet up with the team beforehand and openly discuss your ideas and wishes.

Afterpains

Afterpains often take new second-time mothers off guard. While they can and do affect first-time new mothers, they are much more common, and stronger, the second time around. They caught me completely by surprise. I remember holding my baby two hours after he was born and begging the midwife for an epidural to cope with the afterpains. I distinctly recall telling her that I would go through a thousand labours, rather than deal with any more afterpains.

So what are afterpains? And why are they usually worse with second babies? Afterpains are the body's way of shrinking the uterus to its pre-pregnancy size after the birth of a baby. And they tend to be stronger after a second baby as the uterus has more contracting to do.

The involuntary uterine contractions generally last for the first two or three days after the birth. Breastfeeding tends to stimulate these contractions and can make them stronger. You may also notice an increased flow of lochia (postnatal bleeding) accompanies afterpains.

Some women don't notice afterpains, some feel them very mildly and some really suffer. Research looking at the effectiveness and safety of different types of pain relief for afterpains has found that non-steroidal anti-inflammatories (NSAIDS) such as aspirin and naproxen are more effective than paracetamol and safer than codeine-based medicines which can be dangerous for babies when breastfeeding, due to something known as codeine toxicity.[18] You may also find that a hot-water bottle or heat pack helps to relieve the pain somewhat, and some mothers find that a TENS machine can help too (you may have used one in labour). You can also use any relaxation techniques you learned for labour to help you through afterpains.

Healing from the birth . . . and taking care of two children

There is a bit of a misconception that it is easier to get back to normal after the birth, if the birth was a natural, vaginal one, rather than a C-section. My second birth was quick and straightforward and yet I struggled to walk for at least two days afterwards. I also struggled with horrendous afterpains. C-sections, being major abdominal surgery, obviously need plenty of time to heal from. But no matter how your baby is born, you need to understand that your body has been through a lot and you won't be able to just 'ping' back to normal a day or so later with your firstborn and new baby.

New mothers need time to rest. Don't try to be Superwoman and rush things. That isn't good for your firstborn, your newborn or for you. Plan for somebody to take care of you for at least a week, or preferably two, as a minimum. Meal prep as much as you can before the birth, ask visitors to bring a meal, rather than a new-baby gift or make friends with your local takeaway food providers. Hold off visits from people who end up being more of an inconvenience than a help and don't be afraid to ask for help in whatever form you can get it: cooking, cleaning, laundry, holding the baby or entertaining your first-born. It isn't selfish to take care of yourself. Far from it – it's the most important thing you can do as a new mother to two.

Does this mean it's wrong for you to be active and upright as soon as possible? No – that's OK, but only if it feels good for you. If you are feeling great, the worst thing you can do is to lay around if you want to get moving. Just don't push yourself. Chapters 8 and 9 will look in more detail at the immediate days post-birth, particularly your own emotions and managing the early days with two children; any advice I give there is always underpinned by the premise of taking care of yourself first though, which is so important that I've raised the idea here too.

I hope that this chapter has left you feeling more positive about the birth of your second baby. No matter what your experience was like first time around, I'm certain that this birth will be just as positive (if things went well) or much more so (if things didn't go to plan). Preparation and knowledge are vital, no matter what type of birth you are planning. Birth can be empowering and enjoyable, however it happens, so long as you go into it well prepared and well informed.

To help you feel as calm and relaxed as possible during your labour and birth, you will need to make sure that your firstborn is happy and comfortable while it is happening. Once you know that they are OK, you are free to focus on yourself and the new baby, which is exactly why the next chapter explores what to do with number one, while number two arrives – and how to prepare them for it.

Chapter 7

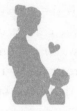

Childcare During Labour and Birth

F or some parents, the decision of who should look after their firstborn while they are giving birth to their second child is an easy one, particularly if they're lucky enough to have helpful family members close by with whom their firstborn has a strong bond. For others, whose family are not local, or those, like myself, who have no close family anywhere, the decision is much harder. Planning childcare for labour plays a huge role in your birth preparation second time around because not only do you need to make sure that your child is calm and happy, you also need to feel confident about your choice too. If not, the anxiety over who is caring for your child can set off the fear-tension-pain cycle (see page 121).

I am an only child and, sadly, my parents (and my husband's) died young, before my own children were born. I have aunts, uncles and cousins, but none very local that we saw regularly, or with whom my son had a strong bond. For this reason, my son had never spent a night away from me until his baby brother was born and not more than a few hours in the daytime. I found the whole idea of childcare for him while I gave birth incredibly stressful, which was one of the main reasons that I decided to plan a home birth. The idea was that I would hopefully go into labour overnight, after my son was tucked up in bed, and he'd wake in the morning to greet the new addition to the family. Fate had other plans. While this is exactly what happened with my fourth baby, I found myself admitted to hospital unexpectedly with my second baby, facing pre-eclampsia and a hospital induction, and we had to make plans quickly. This is one of my biggest regrets surrounding my second birth and the early days with two. I had been so set on a home birth, I hadn't considered what might happen if things took a different turn. As it happens, things worked out OK in the end. Some friends we had made at antenatal classes the first time around offered to have our son overnight. However, it wasn't what I'd planned and I had no time to prepare my son or to make that night easier for him or, indeed, for those caring for him. And still, to this day, I don't know if he was OK; I didn't want to ask our friends, and I doubt they would have told me honestly if he had sobbed all night. So if I could give one piece of advice concerning childcare during labour, it would be to plan and prepare for every eventuality. A back-up plan (and perhaps even a back-up back-up plan) is as important as your main plan.

What are your options?

You may already have a good idea of who you want to care for your child while you are in labour, which is great. I would still recommend, however, that you have a back-up plan or two options from this list, should your first plan unexpectedly not work out. Here are your main options:

- Your firstborn's grandparents

- Your own or your partner's siblings

- Other family members, such as your aunts, uncles and cousins

- Your friends – either from before you had children or new ones you made at antenatal or baby groups

- Neighbours, who could pop round and care for your child or take them in if needed

- Childcare professionals you already know – for instance, your firstborn's childminder, nanny or a nursery worker who may be prepared to help overnight, in your home or their own

- Childcare professionals who offer emergency, ad-hoc childcare; some agencies will offer day nannies or similar, who can be booked for one-off care

- Your partner – some mothers decide to go to hospital alone or with a friend or family member, so that their partner can stay with their firstborn

- A home birth – the idea here is that your child may sleep through the birth or go about their normal daily routine, perhaps with your partner caring for them or a friend or family member

I spoke to some mothers about the childcare plans they made for their firstborns while they were giving birth to their second baby. Here's what they told me:

> Our home birth was perfect for us, as we do not have any childcare near to us and it meant we could stay at home and not disturb the eldest from his routine.

My mum came around and slept over at our house. She looked after my son in the early stages of labour and did the regular preschool run and cooked him dinner. Later, when things picked up, she popped him to bed and my husband and I went to the hospital. We were home with the new baby the next lunchtime!

My friend came and took our daughter back to her house when I realised I was in labour. My daughter is friends with her daughter (in fact, we met at the same antenatal class), and she was really excited about her first sleepover with her friend. So when the time came, she wasn't worried about me being in labour, just excited to go to her friend's house. It worked really well.

We had a home birth, as we had for our eldest, and had involved him in the planning of it, some of the midwife visits and preparation of the lounge for the pool, etc. He was in the house with my mum during my labour and came in and out to see me, including twenty minutes before his little sister was born.

My eldest stayed overnight at another member of our family's home during the birth and the next night, so we could get through the first night at home with our baby and then introduce them to each other the next day on our eldest's terms.

My mum came to stay with us for a week from my due date. Luckily the baby arrived on the fifth day after she had arrived. We left our son with his grandma, while we went off to the hospital. It worked really well, but I don't know what I would have done if the baby had arrived earlier or later!

I have never actually heard a story where things didn't seem to miraculously work out OK in the end – as in Nicola's case, below. I think, in part, because nature is so clever. If mothers-to-be are stressed because of the lack of childcare for their firstborn, labour is inhibited from starting, or progressing, until their child is safe and cared for, allowing them to focus on giving birth again. This makes complete sense when you think back to the hormones involved in the fear-tension-pain cycle and the inhibitory effect cortisol, the stress hormone, has upon oxytocin, the hormone of labour. Nevertheless, it's still worth having a back-up plan.

Nicola's story

I was really concerned about who would care for my eldest son when I went into labour with my second. Both of my parents have passed away, my husband's father is also no longer with us and his mum has dementia and lives in a residential home. I have a sister who lives ten minutes away, but she doesn't drive, has a nine-year-old child and isn't particularly reliable. I have an amazing sister-in-law, who made herself as available as possible, but she works shifts, so couldn't be fully 'on call'. Thankfully, my son's childminder offered to have our son, day or night, if needed.

However, at week forty-one of my pregnancy, all help suddenly disappeared. My sister-in-law and childminder went away and, as I said, I couldn't rely on my sister. I was panicking that I would be alone during my labour while my husband cared for our son. We had thought about a home birth but dismissed it, and I began to regret that decision. I know it was hormones, but I felt so sad that I didn't have any support and felt somewhat let down and abandoned. I cried so much that I felt no one was there for us.

Fortunately, the baby must have sensed my panic as he held on for another eight days until everyone was back home. Plus, conveniently he arrived during the day, while my eldest boy was in childcare!

Juliet's story is another great example of how things tend to simply work out on the day, and the remarkable ability of the human body to know when it's 'safe' for labour to begin. Once again though, the more options you have, the less stress you will put yourself through if plans fall through, or don't quite work out closer to the time.

Juliet's story

When pregnant, I worried a lot about what would happen to my daughter when I went into labour. So much so that I found it hard to imagine beyond going into labour and having a new baby – it really preoccupied and stressed me more than I imagined it would.

Neither my own family nor my husband's live nearby. Friends offered to help out, but we were new to the area and only knew them through having children, so though their offers were kind I didn't really feel I could take them up on them. They had children of their own to look after; plus, I was in labour for twenty-nine hours with my first, and I'm pretty sure their offers of help only meant an emergency hour here or there, not the long haul. Besides, I didn't think my daughter would be happy in that situation.

We decided that my mum was the best person to look after my daughter as they knew each other well and I knew I'd relax if that was the case. The problem was that my mum lives an hour and a half away and doesn't drive. Having her come and stay with us for the last few weeks of pregnancy wasn't feasible as I was sleeping so badly that my husband and I were sleeping separately, and my husband was using the spare room. When we slept together, I slept even worse, and I'd have been furious if that had zapped my energy for labour. I also didn't like the idea of being in early labour at home with my mum around – I know some people want their mothers there, but I think mine would have annoyed me! And I really wanted to do some of the labour at home if I could, as with my first, I'd been induced and had the whole labour in hospital, and I hoped the second labour would be more natural.

So we concluded that we'd find a way to get my mum down when I went into labour. We thought about my husband driving to get her, but with a three-hour round trip, we worried he might miss the birth if things happened very quickly (wishful thinking!). We finally decided that we'd pay for a taxi, even though it would cost about £150. It was cheaper than a hotel room for her for nights on end.

But even knowing this plan was in place, I fretted right until the last minute about my daughter. If something went wrong and my mum couldn't make it, there was no way I wanted my little girl to be with someone she wasn't happy with. I had never spent a night away from her, and I didn't want to make it even more traumatic than it was going to be. On the other hand, the thought of going through labour without my husband (if he had to stay with my daughter) terrified me.

A couple of days past my due date I had some twinges and thought my waters had started to break, but I wasn't sure. My daughter was at nursery and my husband was working from home, so we went over to the hospital to be checked over. Though the twinges got a bit worse, I still wasn't sure. But as soon as the midwife examined me and confirmed my waters had broken, my husband whipped out his phone, rang my mum and booked and paid for her taxi.

The midwife sent us home. My husband picked up my daughter and I made her tea and put her to bed. Things were moving very slowly. I know that I didn't properly relax into it until I heard my mum arrive. She popped her head into the living room, where I was on my ball, and then she left us to it as my husband had asked her to. She went to the spare room to watch TV and it was then that I really believed my daughter was going to be OK and well looked after; labour really ramped up then. We ended up going back to hospital at 10pm that night and I was 4cm dilated, even though just before my mum arrived I'd chatted to a midwife who had estimated I wouldn't need to go in until the next day as things were going so slowly. I really think the relief of knowing my daughter was OK is what made me let go and let things start to happen.

I wonder if it would have been a much, much faster labour if my mum lived five minutes away!

Planning a home birth instead of childcare

For many parents, the idea of a home birth seems the perfect childcare solution. In my years of working as a doula, I think I only attended one home birth with a second baby when the firstborn wasn't asleep in bed during the labour and birth. Most second-time mothers planning a home birth tend to labour at night. They tuck their child up in bed and then relax, feeling safe and calm, which aids the progression of labour. Usually, second babies would arrive in the early hours of the morning, giving the new second-time-parents a couple of hours to bond with their new arrival, before their older child woke up to meet their new sibling at breakfast.

While this is how most second births happen at home, it isn't always the case. Like my second birth, some end up transferring to hospital (either before labour starts or during) and some happen in the daytime when the firstborn is wide awake. This is why you need to plan for all eventualities.

Labour and birth with your firstborn present

There is a strange taboo in our society surrounding birth. We tend to shield children from it. In many other cultures, however, birth is a part of everyday life. It is not something to be hidden or kept behind closed hospital doors. Older siblings often play an active role in the arrival of their new brother or sister. I wanted the latter for my own children and was happy for them to witness their siblings being born.

If you think that you would like your firstborn to be involved in the arrival of your second baby, it is vital that you prepare them for what they will see and hear. Birth is not scary when you understand what is going on, but without that understanding it can be terrifying for young children. The groans, humming, huffing and puffing and occasional yelling and swearing sounds that are part of the birth soundtrack are natural and nothing to be feared, but children need to understand this. Similarly, birth is bloody and messy. For young children, blood tends to be a sign of illness and pain; they don't necessarily understand that it's not dangerous that Mum is bleeding. Also, newborn babies can be very blue and very squished with strange-shaped heads and umbilical cords can look like something from an alien movie. These things can all scare young children and if your firstborn is frightened, you will pick up on their anxiety.

The answer to this is prepare, prepare, prepare. Watch as

many films about giving birth as you can with your child. Explain to them why you may make certain noises, explain what the blood is from and why it's there and explain what they can expect their new sibling to look like when they are born. You should also explain the medical equipment that they are likely to see – things like sonicaids, entonox (gas and air) canisters and baby-resuscitation equipment – and what the midwives will be doing on the day or night. The more you educate and inform, the less scared your child will be.

If your child isn't old enough to understand all of this, then I think you need to make a call as to whether it is the right environment for them to be in. If they are very young and it's not possible to explain to them about normal, natural birth and all that accompanies it, then at the very least you need to have another adult with them throughout the labour and birth, whose sole job is to take care of them, while somebody else takes care of you. This is the role I often fulfilled when working as a doula. I would be there to take care of the firstborn child almost exclusively, while the partner focused on Mum; or, more often, I would focus on supporting the mum, allowing the partner to focus on their firstborn child.

What if you don't want your child there – or they don't want to be there?

Although I didn't end up having a home birth with my second, my third and fourth children were born at home. My fourth arrived following a very quick labour, while the other three were asleep. However, my third baby arrived in the daytime, while his siblings were wide awake. I had wonderful visions of labouring with my sons around me. I wanted them to witness their sibling being born and I wanted them to grow up knowing that birth was normal and natural and nothing to be afraid of. When the day came, they were excited and relaxed. Not a sniff of fear. But what I hadn't anticipated in all our preparation was how utterly unable I would be to labour with my young children around me. I found myself completely incapable of switching off from 'Mummy mode' and relaxing into 'birth mode'. The two did not go well together. In the end, we had to phone a friend and ask her to take the boys to her house for the afternoon. Within thirty minutes of them leaving (and the house becoming significantly quieter), my labour ramped up a gear and my son was born in the birth pool around two hours later. My friend bought the boys home around an hour after their brother arrived. Despite my plan to have my children with me throughout the birth, I really don't think I could ever have switched off enough for it to have gone well.

Similarly, I've been at second-time home births where dads have had to take firstborns out for the day, because they have struggled to cope with all the new people in their house or seeing Mum in labour. This is not a good introduction to life as a new big brother or sister, so having a back-up plan in place, for this eventuality is important.

Of course, this may not happen. You may labour during the night, while your firstborn sleeps, or you may labour in the day, while your firstborn holds your hand helping you to relax, enjoying every minute of watching the new baby arrive. Just like Amy's story below.

Amy's story

I felt very keenly that I wanted my three-year-old daughter to be around when her baby sibling was born. We considered the option of her going to stay with friends or family, but felt that returning home to find a new baby would be too much of a shock for her; she might feel usurped, and we were concerned it could hinder the sibling bonding process.

My husband and I went over and over our options for what to do with her while I was in labour. As we were planning on a home birth, we decided to simply keep her at home with us. We had a list of five very close friends who live near us who said they'd be happy to come by the house and play with her or keep her company, so that my husband could support me and not be distracted. In the week running up to the birth, I had a few false starts, and we had them all on high alert almost daily!

But in the end, fortunately, I went into labour in the evening once my eldest was safely tucked up in bed. She did wake up briefly while I was in the early stages of my contractions, but my husband took her back to bed, and she happily went back to sleep. What was wonderful was that I delivered our baby girl in a pool in our kitchen at around 2 a.m. Our eldest woke up a few minutes later and wandered down the hall into the kitchen to see what was happening.

The expression on her face when she saw me in the water cradling her newborn sister is one I'll remember for ever. She was so delighted; it was perfect. Fortunately, the midwives were on the ball enough to capture the moment on camera, and we have this lovely picture of our new family together, all with huge smiles on our faces.

Our eldest stayed up to 'help' our wonderful midwives measure her new little sister. She was even fascinated by the placenta which the midwives showed her. Eventually, she went back to bed, and after the midwives left, my husband and I were left to marvel at our new addition.

Preparing your firstborn for what will happen when you are in labour

This is a little like preparing them for the arrival of the new baby. Young children struggle with abstract and hypothetical thinking and so, unless your children are older (five years and upwards), it's unlikely that they will really grasp what is about to happen, or truly understand the impact it might have on them.

If your firstborn is older, then the best preparation is to sit down with them and talk through what will happen and when, making sure that you answer any questions they may have. Ask them if they can think of anything that they would like to take (if they will be staying elsewhere), or if there is anything they would like you to leave with them, if they are staying at home. Some children, for instance, like to have a photo of their parents with them or an item of Mum's clothing, with her scent on it, to snuggle up to at night.

If your age gap is smaller and your firstborn is still a toddler, or of preschool age, then be prepared that any explanations may not be entirely effective. Focus on trying to make sure that they are as comfortable as possible with the person who will be caring for them. A practice run is a great idea, as this can show up any potential problems while you are still around to step in and help, rather than leaving them until the day, when there is little to nothing you can do. Make sure that whoever will be caring for your child knows any routines they have, particularly around sleep. Involving the adult who will be looking after your child in one or more bedtime routines in the run-up to the baby's arrival can be really helpful, not just so that the adult knows what happens, how and when, but so that your firstborn becomes used to them being around to settle them at bedtime. Also, think about any comfort items that your child may find helpful in your absence, such as sleeping with a blanket or pillow from your bed, or simply making sure they have their favourite teddy with them. Another great idea is to take photos of your child with the adult who will be caring for them, particularly at different points during the day and night. If your child will be going to a different house, then take photos of the house and the room your child will be sleeping in. Print these out and use them to make a small scrapbook, making up a story that you can share with your child in the weeks before the new baby is due.

I would also recommend that you write a 'While I'm Giving Birth Plan' for your firstborn. Like your birth plan, this is a way to write down anything that is important to you or your child, so that the adult caring for them has a written record of important points, rather than trying to remember everything, or you or your partner having to try to remind them when you're in labour and have other things on your mind. These are some things you may want to put in this plan:

- The times your child usually sleeps

- What you do in their bedtime routine (including any favourite bedtime books)

- The times your child usually eats

- What food your child reliably eats (and what they really hate)

- What special comfort objects your child has (and what their names are)

- Any activities, games or television programmes your child particularly enjoys

- A reminder of timings of any groups they attend, or school pick-up and drop-off times

- For childcare staff, a reminder of any allergies, or medical needs

When you pack your hospital bag or arrange your home-birth kit (I usually recommend doing both at around thirty-six weeks) you should also pack your child a bag with anything they may need while you're in labour, if they're going to be cared for by somebody else. Pack the bag with enough for two days, even if you're planning for a natural birth or home birth. Don't forget to put a copy of the 'While I'm Giving Birth Plan' into the bag too, even if you have previously given the carer a copy. Finally, consider sending them with some of their favourite snacks and a bottle or cup from home, so that they have small items of security with them, as well as any comfort objects, and consider packing a few small toys and books too.

When should you call in childcare or drop your child off?

The decision of when to call in your childcare or drop your child off is really a personal one. Some parents prefer their child to be with them until the very last minute, just before they leave for hospital or call the midwives out for a home birth. Others prefer to get their firstborn settled in the early stages, allowing them to focus on labouring without worrying about their child. There really is no right or wrong answer here. Calling a little later avoids the repeat 'false alarms' that can happen second-time around; however, there is also a risk that you may end up accidentally leaving things too late. Remember, the time that you call must take into consideration how close the carer is to your home. If they are in the same street as you and you've called them earlier to put them on standby, then you really can wait until the last minute. If they are an hour or more away, then calling earlier and asking if they would perhaps wait in another room (unless you want them around you) or go out locally or even go to sleep if it's night-time, is probably sensible. Talking through different scenarios with them in advance and weighing up what you think would be best for both you and your child is the way to go.

One of the secrets to the easiest birth for you and smoothest transition in the first day or two for your firstborn is undoubtedly how you plan for childcare during labour. The best plans are those that cover all eventualities and remain flexible, but are, at the same time, well thought out and rehearsed. When the big day arrives, this planning allows you to relax and concentrate on giving birth, safe in the knowledge that your firstborn is happy and well cared for.

Chapter 8

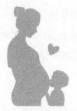

The Baby's Here!
And So Is the Guilt

I am aware that this chapter (and indeed, the next three) might make for uncomfortable reading. My intention is not to scare anybody or portray life with two children in a negative light. I hope, however, that in being honest and talking about topics and feelings which so often seem to be taboo, I will be able to help you to feel more confident and at peace about life with two children. Of course, some of you might struggle to identify with some of the more upsetting feelings that I write about, which is brilliant! But others will find the transition tougher. And this chapter is written predominantly with you in mind. I want to bring things out into the open and help new second-time parents to realise that what they are feeling is OK. It's common, it's normal and it doesn't make you a bad or ungrateful parent. Most importantly, I want to reassure you that things will improve.

It's strange for me writing this chapter. While I remember

the feelings of doubt, guilt, grief and regret quite vividly, they also seem like a lifetime ago to me now, even though I'm only fourteen years on from the birth of my second child. I look back now and wish I could give myself a hug, tell myself that everything will be OK and that I won't feel bad for ever. But instead, I'd like to pass that virtual hug along to you instead.

Maternal guilt

One of the toughest things about becoming a mother for the first time is learning to cope with feeling guilty. We feel guilty if we don't 'love every minute' (nobody does, by the way), we feel guilty if we lose our temper (which we all do), we feel guilty when we desperately need a break from our children, we feel guilty about the parenting choices we make or those that were made for us and we feel guilty about not doing enough self-care. We just can't win. Physical exhaustion and sleep deprivation aside, the guilt must be one of the worst things about new motherhood. First-time mother guilt is hard, really hard. And the second time around, you have the same guilt as the first time and so much more. The good news though, is that it is normal. And knowing this helped me to feel so much better. It didn't lift the guilt any quicker, but taking away the nagging self-doubt made it much easier to cope with.

This chapter will look at some of the most common feelings of guilt that second-time mothers experience and how to move forwards.

Turning your firstborn's world upside down

The disruption another baby brings to your firstborn's life has already been discussed, but I wanted to bring it up again here.

Sadly, those feelings of guilt commonly increase when the new baby arrives. For some, the new wave of guilt hits the minute they leave their firstborn to give birth to a new baby. For others, it doesn't hit until a few weeks, or even months, down the line. I have never met a mother who didn't feel guilty about changing her firstborn's world, though.

I spoke to some second-time mothers and asked them when the feelings of guilt for changing their firstborn's world hit them. This is what they told me:

The guilt I felt was incredible. I was in hospital for a week. This was so hard as my four-year-old daughter had never been away from me for more than two nights (and even then, it was only once). The first night was the worst: she screamed the entire hospital down leaving me, even before the baby was born. It certainly accentuated all the Mum guilt about having another baby! However, my partner was really supportive to her through this; he gave her treats, but also talked to her as a human with real feelings and explained properly why Mummy had to be there.

I remember my first night in hospital after the birth of my second child so well. My first child was just over two and a half years old at this point and the previous few months with her had been so much fun. We would do lots of activities together and have long conversations about things. And suddenly, there I was, with a tiny, helpless baby lying next to me in the plastic hospital crib, looking so fragile. Every time I was about to go off to sleep, he would make a tiny crying sound. I was so tired after a previous sleepless night giving birth to him, longing for some sleep, and missing my daughter so much. I wanted to hold my little son, but I also just needed to sleep. I would pick him up and sit there upright in my bed, scared I would fall asleep with him in my arms. This made me miss my daughter even more, as she would often spend part of the night sleeping in my arms. I remember being full of feelings: guilty for being away from my daughter, and guilty for not enjoying this first night with my son more. I had so been looking forward to meeting him and falling in love with him, and I had not been expecting all the other feelings. It was an incredibly conflicting and lonely moment.

My son was born nine days before my daughter turned one. She was still a baby herself and for three quarters of her life I'd been pregnant and dealing with morning sickness and tiredness. My daughter wasn't walking when my second baby was born, so I had two babies to carry, essentially. My daughter wouldn't hug or cuddle me for about a week after getting home with my son from hospital; it was like her affection was on strike and it was heartbreaking. I just wanted to sit and cuddle and bond with my new son, but felt guilty and had to cut time with him to make time for her, when she needed it. I constantly felt I was being 50 per cent of the mum they each needed.

When your firstborn suddenly seems huge

I remember the sense of shock I felt when I held my second baby for the first time. My babies are huge at birth (ten and eleven pounders), but he felt so very tiny. Realising how tiny he was made me cry because it reminded me that my firstborn was not a baby any more. My older son, even though he was only fifteen months, felt huge. Suddenly, it seemed like I had missed a chunk of his life somehow. The feel of a tiny new baby in my arms made me mourn a little for the baby that my firstborn had been. In turn, that made me reminisce about the early days as a brand-new mother – just myself, my firstborn son and my husband, which made me realise that our little family of three no longer existed.

I thought I was insane for mourning my firstborn's baby-hood, when he was alive and well and a thriving toddler, until I spoke to more second-time mothers and realised that many had felt the same. The feeling didn't last for long because life as a family of four quickly became the new normal. I also spent several hours looking at my firstborn's baby photos, looking for similarities and differences between him and his new brother, which helped to allay my craving for my firstborn as a baby.

Not having the time to bond with the new baby

The first few weeks, or even months, of life with a baby and a toddler felt very much focused on my older son. We went to his playgroups, met with his friends and went for days out to entertain him. Days revolved around my firstborn's mealtimes and nap times, while my second-born either slept on me in a sling or in his Moses basket in our living room, in between some snatched time for breastfeeds. Once my firstborn had gone to bed, I would pick up my new baby for what felt like the first time that day. Of course, I had picked him up several times in the day, but those felt very functional: a quick feed, a hasty nappy change and so on. I didn't feel like I had any time in the day to just cuddle him and get to know him. I felt so guilty that I was depriving him of my full attention and inhibiting bonding in some way. The truth was, he was very settled, calm, well-fed, clean and content, but I felt like I should be giving him more.

I felt sad that I wasn't going to any baby groups with my new son. Instead, he was being dragged along to toddler music classes and the like. I finally felt the guilt ease a little, when I booked us into baby massage classes at around six weeks. My older son spent a few hours with a childminder (who he loved, which helped to ease any potential guilt there) and I could finally spend time one-to-one focusing solely on my new baby. Baby massage added to this experience, as we spent an hour each week looking into each other's eyes and releasing lots of oxytocin with the skin-to-skin touch. I would recommend that you don't worry about going to any baby classes or groups with the new baby, but if you can, try to get to a baby massage class or two. It really does help with bonding and feeling less guilty about the time they spend strapped on your chest in a carrier or rather ignored in a crib.

Giving your baby attention in front of your firstborn

The irony was that while I felt guilty for not spending enough quality time bonding with my new baby, if I did manage to do so, then I immediately felt guilty if this was in front of my firstborn. This is so common among second-time mothers I have spoken to. So many tell me that they feel guilty for holding and cuddling their new baby if their older child is in the same room. They worry about upsetting their older child's feelings or somehow making them feel less loved.

Thankfully, this feeling wore off quite quickly, entirely of its own accord, as it does with most mothers. But until it did, I took solace in the night feeds which, when my firstborn was safely tucked up asleep, felt like our stolen secret – an illicit affair, in a way. As exhausted as I was, I would savour the quiet and still night to hold and cuddle and gaze at my new baby as he fed, safe in the knowledge that my firstborn was fast asleep and would not witness my display of love towards another. My second baby slept through the night freakishly early, at around four months, and I still remember how sad I was to lose our special time together. I found myself wishing that he would wake again, which was ironic, considering I had been ecstatic when my firstborn had started to sleep through the night.

Not doing the same for your new baby as you did for your first

One form of guilt that lasted a long time (and still hasn't completely gone, if I'm honest) came from the inability to do with your second-born what you did with your first. My first baby had homemade organic, steamed vegetables for weaning. My second-born was weaned on family leftovers and more jars of baby food than I'd care to admit. My firstborn had beautiful, immaculate clothing, bought specially for him, while at least half of my second-born's wardrobe was hand-me-downs, as were most of the equipment he used and toys he played with. During my first pregnancy, I lovingly filled in a baby diary and journal. I could tell you exactly when my son said his first word and took his first step. I can't actually tell you what my second baby's first word was, let alone when he said it, and I only know when he began walking because we took him to get some first walker shoes fitted the next day and the shoe shop took a photograph and dated it.

I spent hours reading to my firstborn, teaching him baby sign language, singing with him and going to every baby group possible. But perhaps most telling of all is the wall of professional baby photos we had taken when our firstborn was three months old. They cost the equivalent of a foreign holiday (we justified their purchase by the fact that we weren't going away that year). They hung, pride of place, in beautiful frames in our living room, whereas there were only a couple of photos of my second-born in cheap supermarket photo frames. We didn't have the same disposable income, the inclination or the space to repeat the ridiculously overpriced photo package again. The only saving grace as my second son gets older and asks where all his baby photos are, is that I have barely any of his younger brother and none at all of his sister, our fourth born.

Sometimes I still feel a little guilty over not giving my children the same in their babyhood, but in my more rational moments, I really don't think it matters. The only people who remember life before two children now are myself and my husband. My second-born didn't know what he had missed and certainly didn't suffer because of it. So in wistful moments, I remind myself that it really doesn't matter, not to them anyway.

Breastfeeding guilt

Something I come across a lot among second-time mothers is breastfeeding guilt. They feel guilty if they didn't manage to breastfeed with their first baby but were successful the second time around; or if they breastfed their first, but didn't manage to feed their second-born; or if they fed them for differing lengths. Finally, they feel guilty for feeling the need to wean their firstborn, either during pregnancy or shortly after their second baby arrives if they had planned to tandem feed, but found it didn't work out for them.

There is no doubt that breastfeeding is the norm for our species and optimum for health. However, that doesn't mean that formula milk is the food of the devil. Our society needs to invest more in breastfeeding, in improved support, better knowledge among health-care professionals and greater training in spotting tongue tie. So if your breastfeeding journey didn't work out how you had hoped, whether it was with your first or second baby, or perhaps both, it's so important that you

realise you didn't fail at anything. Try to be at x
knowledge that you did what you could, and you
giving, your very best to your baby. I have breastfe
children for hugely varying lengths, from six weeks,
years. None of them, as teenagers, has the faintest inter
how they were fed as a baby. Any time I spent beating my x
up about the different ways they were fed has had no impact
on how they feel about me, or their upbringing.

Feeling you're never quite meeting anybody's needs

Too many mothers feel as if they are failing. We are our own
harshest critics – more so than those in any other occupation.

I remember the days when my baby and toddler cried in
unison; there were a few when I joined them too. I remember
the days when I went to bed, with a messy house and a frozen
pizza hastily thrown in the oven, thinking, 'I'm just no good
at this, I'm barely surviving.' But survive we did; we made it
through the day, the next day and the next. All in one piece.
So my mantra on the bad days was 'Nobody died, everybody
survived'. Keeping us all alive and healthy became my baseline.
And if I had a really good day, I would give myself a virtual high
five and feel like Supermum. Gradually, the good days became
more and more frequent – although a decade and a half later, I
think there are probably still only 70 per cent Supermum days
to 30 per cent survival days. But I've become less of a self-critic.
I realise that I'm doing my best and that's good enough.

In the early days, I'd really recommend adopting a nobody-
died-everybody-survived mentality, and just see the good days
as a positive and unexpected extra when they happen. It's OK
to just aim for survival.

*

Shauna's story, below, is a great example of the differing forms of guilt so often experienced by mothers in the early days of life with two children.

Shauna's story

When my daughter was born, I felt guilty kissing and hugging her in front of my son, in case he would get jealous and resentful. But then I also started to worry that I wasn't giving my daughter enough attention and stimulation because the needs of a young toddler are so great. I worried that she wasn't going to develop properly. Mainly though, I worried my son wasn't getting enough attention. He would often try to climb on me, especially when I was breastfeeding, and I felt I was rejecting him because I was worried he'd hurt the baby. In my most sleep-deprived state, I was convinced that I had ruined both their lives by having them close together.

The worst experience was when my son had a febrile seizure, but I didn't hear him fitting straight away because I was putting my daughter to bed. I blamed myself for not being more attentive. Could I have prevented it if I wasn't dividing my attention between two small people? And when my son went to A&E, I was heartbroken I couldn't be in the ambulance to comfort him because I still had to look after my baby girl.

I still feel like it is a daily balancing act to meet both their needs, and new phases in their growth and development bring new challenges. My son, however, clearly loves his sister and, so far, doesn't show any ill feelings towards her and one day he won't remember life without her. But as a mum, the guilt I have felt has been painful and continues to worry me every day.

Hospital stays

I often come across questions from mothers asking how to help their firstborns to cope with hospital stays, whether they need medical attention during their pregnancy or after the birth or their newborn has had a medical problem. As with most maternal guilt, the level felt is usually in proportion with any potential trauma experienced by the firstborn child. While there are some things that you can do to help your firstborn with the tricky transition, if you find yourself in this position, it's just as vital to take care of yourself and your own feelings. Be kind to yourself and try to find a little space to offload and recharge. Don't fight what you're going through; just allow your feelings to be. But do talk to hospital staff about them, as they will have dealt with this sort of situation many times before and can often offer good advice and reassurance.

If you do find yourself having to stay in hospital, either for yourself or your newborn, the following tips can help your firstborn to adjust and cope in your absence:

- Frame a photograph of yourself for your firstborn's bed-side table or windowsill.

- Record a video message for them to play when they miss you.

- Utilise online video messaging services for reading bed-time stories and blowing goodnight kisses at the end of each day.

- Take a special soft blanket with you to the hospital and sleep with it, so it retains your scent (or spray it with your favourite perfume), take a photo or video of yourself with it and then send it home to be with your child, for them to cuddle when they can't have you.

- If your child visits you in hospital, try to meet with them in the hospital garden or cafeteria if there is one. Meeting on less medical territory (even if you're wheeled down in a wheelchair) might help them to feel less afraid.

- Make sure that whoever cares for your child sticks to any regular schedules that they have, including eating and bedtime routines. Regularity and a sense of normality can really help them in your absence.

- Be prepared for your child to have big feelings. They may shun your attention, they may not stop crying, they may become very clingy with you. These are all totally normal reactions. They will pass, but often this will take longer than you would expect – sometimes several weeks or even months after you've returned home. Don't try to rush them through this stage. Allow them to be angry, upset, frustrated and sad. Don't punish them for their feelings or try to reward them to 'behave'. Just let them be. Offer comfort, listening and be patient.

In the story below, Hannah, talks about the arrival of her second baby, her unexpected stay in the neonatal intensive care unit (NICU) and the guilt she felt towards her firstborn, even though things turned out OK in the end.

Hannah's story

With my second son it had never even occurred to me that I'd stay in hospital for more than a day or two after the birth. My first birth had been positive and straightforward and, other than breastfeeding being a steep learning curve, everything had been quite textbook. I'd expected the same uncomplicated birth and hospital timeframe second time around or, if anything, an even smoother/quicker experience.

However, the birth of my second son was traumatic and within a few hours of his birth he was in NICU being prodded and tested due to laboured breathing. It took me totally by surprise and I felt hugely underprepared. It was a mix of emotions: worry and disappointment with the birth, happiness to have my baby in any arms, but total shock with the overall experience. I remember crying all the time that this wasn't how it was meant to be and blaming myself that the bad birth had resulted in the complications, so I should have done things differently (this took a long time to shake off – the feeling that I was to blame).

We ended up staying in hospital for six days. I thought I'd traumatised my firstborn for life because he was not happy being home without me. I felt endless guilt as it was the first time I'd left him for more than a night and like a failure for not preparing him for this scenario. This blame and guilt remained with me for months.

I wish someone had told me that the guilt and blame were entirely unnecessary. I now know that my eldest son has no recollection of that time, and no trauma. In fact, he doesn't remember a time before his brother was in his life. They are best friends and enhance each other's lives so much. It was all worth it. However hard it is at the time, it's worth it. A sibling is life's greatest gift and to give that to your firstborn child is a privilege – however rocky the road may initially be.

In her story below, Emily talks about the diagnosis of her son's medical problems during her second pregnancy and the bumpy start they had as a new family of four. Her story is a brilliant example of how to gently guide and support a firstborn child through the arrival of a new baby sibling with medical problems requiring hospitalisation.

Emily's story

Our two-year-old firstborn, Imogen, is a perceptive little girl. Even before her little brother arrived she grasped that big changes were ahead. But none of us was prepared for the news to come. After a routine pregnancy scan, our unborn son, James, was diagnosed with multiple heart defects. Then, at twenty-nine weeks' gestation, we received another blow: I was diagnosed with placental insufficiency. We mentally prepared ourselves for the worst, despite hoping and praying for the best. It was a difficult time, navigating Imogen through the excitement of the baby's arrival, while being hesitant due to the doubt. The pregnancy was understandably hard emotionally, for us all. We had to face a lot of uncertainty and anxiety, we needed to grieve the loss of the healthy wee boy we thought we had, the potential loss of James (both pre- and post-birth) and the lack of normality and challenges we had to face.

Miraculously, we got to thirty-seven weeks of pregnancy and James was delivered via a planned C-section. It was a huge relief and utter joy to see his beautiful, perfect face when he came into the world. I had to leave Imogen for the birth, having not been away from her for more than about seven hours before, which was hard. We told her before going to the hospital that she would get to meet her new baby brother soon. However, we were then informed that she was not allowed to visit James in the NICU. It was difficult explaining to Imogen that her baby brother had arrived, but that she couldn't see him yet. We felt it important that we explained to her, at an age-appropriate level, what was happening, even when things were not looking good. It is likely to be far more upsetting and scary to a child knowing something is wrong, but not knowing what. Imogen got to meet James briefly for the first time when he was six days old, on his way to having open-heart surgery. Instead of getting to bring her new sibling home like other children, she also had to cope with the fact that her mother would not come home for weeks. Not surprisingly, Imogen resented James for this.

We were very fortunate to have my mother-in-law stay in our home to help, especially with Imogen, which provided stability for our daughter, given all the changes that were happening around her. My husband would also spend as much time as he could at home, while juggling work commitments and being there for James and me. My mother-in-law came to the hospital to visit with Imogen every day. It was a trying time, as while Imogen and I were very happy to be reunited, she could end up having major meltdowns. We tackled this by talking about how she was feeling and normalising her emotions, letting her know often how much we loved and missed her. For instance, by saying things like: 'It must be so hard for you not having Mummy home. I miss you heaps too and wish I could be home with you.' Above all, we tried to be as patient as possible with her, understanding that when she 'acted up' it was her way of dealing with big emotions. We would try to offer 'time in' (lots of hugs and comfort) and spend quality time with her whenever possible, and we found that treats and occasional little gifts helped too, to show her that we were thinking of her. She also slept with a photograph of me and my husband next to her bed every night.

When James was transferred to a different hospital, there was no place for me to stay overnight. The first night I walked away was one of the hardest things I have ever had to do. My only consolation was that I was finally going home to my daughter and husband. Imogen and I got to talk more about how hard it had been for her. It felt so good to feel I had my daughter back, even though I had never really lost her.

We finally brought James home when he was six weeks old. This was a huge turning point for Imogen and her relationship with her brother. It felt as if things at last were as they should be. She showed utter adoration for James and became the wonderful, caring big sister we always knew she would be. After the bumpy start, we felt it was important to let her develop her relationship with her brother at her own pace. James is now a healthy, gorgeous wee boy who is thriving – his heart surgery was extremely successful, despite his small size and he is breastfeeding and gaining weight well. He has blown all the health professionals away.

Overcoming the guilt

No matter what is the cause or root of your feelings of guilt, my advice is to remember you're not the first mother to feel this and you definitely won't be the last. The steps below can help you to slowly accept, work with and finally overcome the guilt that a second baby often brings:

- Recognise that what you are feeling is common and normal: you're not alone.

- Accept your feelings. Allow them to exist. Don't think that feeling this way is wrong.

- Be kind to yourself. Remember, it's OK if all you did today was survive.

- Remind yourself that images of family life you see on the internet or even in real life are just snippets (well-edited snippets, if they're on social media). They represent other families at their best; don't compare your worst to their best!

- Try to find just five or ten minutes per day to unwind. I don't mean taking time away from your children (unless you want to), but time to just sit and focus on breathing, listening to a mindfulness recording or similar, just to unload your head a little each day.

- Talk to other second-time mothers. Hearing others share their gritty feelings can help you to feel less alone and more sane.

- Don't feel the need to be Supermum. Taking care of a child and a new baby is enough. It's OK if your house is messy and you're eating frozen meals. It's also OK to use the television as a babysitter sometimes, when you are finding things overwhelming.

- Do talk with your health visitor or doctor if your feelings are becoming hard for you to handle, or if you think you may be developing anxiety or depression.

I'd like to end this chapter with a quote by the American actress Jennifer Edwards:

The beauty of life is, while we cannot undo what is done, we can see it, understand it, learn from it and change, so that every new moment is spent not in regret, guilt, fear or anger, but in wisdom, understanding and love.

Ultimately, when you really think about it – it is always love underpinning second-baby guilt: love for your firstborn and love for your new baby. Focus on the fact that these feelings are caused by the purest and most valuable emotion of all. The fact that you feel guilt, shows how much you love your family and, in turn, what a great mother you are, even if you don't feel like it right now.

Chapter 9

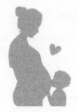

Beautiful Chaos: the Early Days with Two

D o you remember the first day home with your first baby? I remember coming home from hospital, my husband carrying my son into our home in his new car seat and gently putting it down on our living-room floor. We both sat on the sofa and stared at our newborn son in complete silence. One of us – I'm not sure who, but it doesn't matter because we were thinking exactly the same thing – said, 'What do we do now?' I remember vividly that mix of excitement, confusion and trepidation. As it happens, what we did next was to curl up on the sofa and go to sleep, after transferring the baby into his new Moses basket. We all slept for two solid hours, catching up on the lost sleep from the previous crazy day and night.

The first day with your second-born is usually slightly less daunting than the first day with your first baby. You know how to change a nappy, hold a baby, bathe them and what to do when they cry. Yet, you have the added complexity of slotting this new life into a family with another child to care for.

Coming home from hospital with my second baby looked very different. I arrived home to a living room cluttered with toys, a huge mountain of dirty washing that needed attention, a Moses basket that was housing several wooden trains and metal cars and a toddler eager to climb into my lap and pat his new baby brother in a less than gentle way. This all played out to the theme tune of 'Thomas the Tank Engine', blaring from the TV. The term 'beautiful chaos' came to mind. And it's a phrase I think is very fitting for the early days with two young children. There are distinct moments of beauty (the first time your two babies meet face to face), but many, many moments of chaos. At first, you may be tempted to fight the chaos, to try to replicate the calm and quiet of the early post-natal days with your firstborn. I did too. Ultimately, though, I learned to embrace our new normal. You can never reproduce life with one baby, when you already have another. Things will be busier, louder, crazier and, often, more stressful, but that doesn't mean that they are wrong. And it certainly doesn't mean that they are wrong for the new baby either. I don't think it is any coincidence that second babies are usually easier in terms of temperament and sleep – because they are used to fitting in with an already established life, rather than having life revolve around them. If you can surf the turmoil in the early days, things will almost certainly be easier for it over the coming weeks, months and years.

This chapter covers some of the most common questions and concerns that parents have in the early days at home with a second baby, and some tips to survive the beautiful chaos that is now your life.

Healing after the birth

First time around, you had the benefit of being able to 'sleep when the baby sleeps' – that deeply irritating, yet appropriate advice. In the early days with my first baby, particularly when my partner was back at work and I was alone with him, I did make full use of his naps and often slept too. However, I discovered very early on that 'sleep when the baby sleeps' definitely doesn't apply to second babies. When the baby slept, if my toddler didn't wake him up (which occurred often, something we'll look at later), he would desperately want me to play with him. Baby naps are a great opportunity to reconnect with your firstborn, one to one, and try to rebuild some of the connection that may have been lost during the pregnancy and birth and immediate postnatal period. And if I wasn't playing, I felt I really had to do some housework, prepare lunch for us or think about dinner. Often, we were running off to different playgroups too.

Postnatal healing, or rather the opportunity for it, is definitely more of a challenge second time around, however more realistic expectations and the coping strategies that you have from first time around often make it easier, as these mums found:

> I felt much better the second time around as the newborn stage wasn't as much of a shock.

> I was much more organised second time. I worked out a real plan for making food and managed to fit in micro naps when both children were sleeping.

Nevertheless, and as I've already said, you really need to resist the temptation to be Supermum. Taking enough time to heal from the birth, particularly if you had a C-section or perineal stitches, is important. You may feel that you are neglecting your older child by not getting up and playing with them, or doing nursery or school runs, but actually, by resting in the short term, you are actually helping them more in the long run. If you don't try to rest and give your body the opportunity to heal, there is a good chance you will find yourself with a scar rupture, infection or other unpleasant side effect, which could result in hospitalisation and more time away.

To get back to normal quicker, you need to work out a way to rest in the early days. For me, my partner took more time off from work the second time than he had with our firstborn – three weeks, as opposed to two. It was a struggle financially, but so helpful, as it allowed me to really focus on healing before he had to go back to work and leave me flying solo. If you don't have a partner, or it's not possible for them to take much time off work, you really must find a way to get some practical, hands-on help, whether that's your parents, parents-in-law, another family member, a friend, or paid-for help, such as a postnatal doula or mother's help. Never under-estimate how important your healing is and don't feel guilty for needing to sleep in the early days, even if your firstborn is desperate to play, because taking care of yourself means taking care of them too.

Babymooning with two

The early days at home are also about bonding with your new baby. Your babymoon will undoubtedly look different second-time around, but that doesn't mean that bonding is any less important. Perhaps the most important piece of advice I can give you is to not rush yourself into feeling bonded with your new baby. You will have less time to dote on your newborn, and so it makes sense that it may take longer for you to fall in love with them. I wish somebody had told me this in the early days of life with two.

In the early days, it can feel very much as though you are robotically going through the motions: feeding, winding, changing nappies, getting to sleep – while also taking care of your firstborn. It would often get to the end of the day and I would think, 'I've held the baby lots today, but I don't feel I've given him any proper attention'. This is where the nights are so perfect. The still, dark quiet, when just the two of you can get to know each other properly, without the busyness of your older chid clambering over you, needing your attention.

One mistake that new families of four often make is for the dad, or partner or other family members to take over most of the parenting of the firstborn child, leaving Mum at home with the baby. This seems to make obvious sense at first, especially if she is breastfeeding. However, in my experience, it's the most common cause of problematic behaviour from the firstborn. What your firstborn needs when a new baby arrives is reassurance that you still love them. To them, love means time – and undivided time and attention at that. While it's certainly easier for other members of your family to take your eldest off to nursery, preschool, school, clubs and the park, leaving you to rest and bond with the baby, there is a real danger that it may make your firstborn feel unconnected to you and pushed out of your affections. If you're feeling up to it, try to make time to nip out quickly, preferably without the baby, for a few minutes per day. Even if it's a nursery or school run, it could make a huge difference to your firstborn. This idea will be picked up again in the next chapter (and some more ideas of what it looks like in practice) because it's so important and so key to the smoothest transition and babymoon possible.

Visitors, midwife and health-visitor check-ups

When your first baby arrives, you are often inundated with visitors, keen to meet the new arrival, soon after the birth. The second time around, however, interest tends to wane a little. Sadly, in our society, there is a special kind of fever-pitched excitement surrounding the birth of a first child, that is never matched by the response to subsequent new arrivals. Congratulations and visitors can be slower to arrive and thinner on the ground. It can be hard to not take this seeming lack of interest personally. I remember thinking, 'Do they think my new son is not as important as my other one?' and feeling deeply hurt that fewer people seemed to want to meet him. It also made *me* feel less special and took some of the edge off the new-mother celebration. The more mothers I spoke to, however, the more I realised that this scenario was commonplace. So if you find yourself in this situation, don't take it as an indication that friends and relatives won't love your new child just as much as your first, or show less interest in them as they grow. And on the positive side, fewer visitors in the early days can make the transition to a new family of four far easier because it gives you time to focus on both of your children, without the routine-busting hustle and bustle that visitors usually bring with them. Savour the lack of visitors rather than mourning it.

On the other hand, if you do find yourself inundated with visitors, don't be afraid to hold them back, or at least ask them to visit at a time that suits you. Spacing them out over several weeks is far better for both children than for all of them to arrive at once. If your older child usually naps at a specific time, ask the visitors to come after the nap has started, or even better, ended, so that they don't disturb their sleep. An overtired and overstimulated child and a house full of visitors, plus a new baby, is a bit of a recipe for disaster. Also, don't be tempted to play the role of the perfect host. I found that visitors viewed me as being more capable as a new second-time mother than they did the first time around. In part, I guess that was true, but it didn't mean that I was feeling up to making food and waiting on them. Ask any visitors to eat before they arrive or, even better, to bring food with them for you to share too. Finally, don't be afraid to ask your visitors to leave, if they are overstimulating your children, particularly your firstborn. It can be really overwhelming for little people to have a house full of people as well as a new baby.

Establishing breastfeeding and entertaining during feeds

No matter how much of a seasoned pro you are, breastfeeding your second baby can be and often is a whole new experience and it can take time to get it established.

All babies are different, as are the situations after giving birth, so allow yourself time to get breastfeeding off to a good start. If you are struggling, in pain or your baby isn't gaining weight or seems unsettled, then regardless of what you think you know from the first time around, call in a breastfeeding counsellor or a lactation consultant to help. Different babies often need different feeding techniques and problems, such as tongue tie and latching problems, can occur second time around, even if breastfeeding was trouble-free the first time.

In the first few weeks and months, you're going to spend a lot of time feeding your newborn, whether you are breastfeeding or bottle-feeding. Some mums can breastfeed on the move with the baby in a sling – wrap slings are usually the favourite style for doing this; if you can, then the sling will be an amazing tool, and don't ever worry about overusing it. But if you need to remain still and focus on your baby to feed, then having some entertainment ideas on hand to occupy your firstborn while you feed is a must. The following can all work well:

- **Enlist your firstborn as a 'special helper'.** Give them a special job to perform each time the baby is due a feed, such as bringing you a fresh muslin, a cushion or a clean nappy and some wipes, to change the baby afterwards.

- **Give your firstborn a realistic baby doll to feed.** Aim to get a doll the same sex as their new sibling and encourage them to breastfeed their baby or give them a doll's bottle at the same time as you bottle-feed their sibling.

- **Create a special feeding basket of toys.** These should be small, quiet toys that don't make a mess, that only come out at feeding time. Good examples of things to include are peg boards, threading-reel sets, Duplo or Lego bricks, jigsaw puzzles, or wooden puzzle boards, water painting mats and magic painting books. Keeping this basket for feed times only preserves the contents' appeal.

- **Embrace the television, tablets and smartphones.** Download and record episodes of your child's favourite programmes for feed times. If you keep the screens off the rest of the day, this makes screen time more interesting during feeds.

- **Listen to audiobooks.** Encourage your firstborn to snuggle up to you and listen to their favourite stories. Or, if you can manage with one hand, read a special book to them during feed times.

- **Feed your firstborn too.** Snacks, lunches and dinners can be timed to fit around the baby's feeds. You can also offer a bottle or cup of milk or a breastfeed (if you're tandem feeding) at the same time as the baby.

I spoke to some mothers about what helped them when it came to feeding the baby in the early days. Here's what they told me:

> I had prepared myself for six weeks of focusing on establishing a successful breastfeeding journey and I knew the difficulties we might have faced. Emotionally, it was difficult as my two-year-old was wondering why I couldn't play as much, but we have made it to nine months breastfeeding so far, and we are finding it easier to deal with.

> Prior to giving birth, I felt as though I had done a really good job in preparing our daughter for the arrival of our second child. We had talked a lot about the baby, but not too much. We had consistently referred to the baby as "our baby" and I had avoided attributing any change in my parenting to being pregnant. Once I came home with the baby, I realised there were lots of things we hadn't, and perhaps couldn't, have prepared for. I wasn't prepared for how upset my daughter would be when she saw me breastfeed the baby, even though she hadn't breastfed for over a year. I think I was hard on myself in those first weeks, expecting myself to cope completely. I found it helpful to name the changes and frustrating feelings we were both experiencing to my daughter. I think it helped us both feel validated.

> For me, one of the most helpful things we did was expressing breast milk and getting the baby used to the bottle from five to six weeks. This was the toughest period for us, as the baby cluster fed for hours on end. Giving him

a bottle in the evening meant that I could put our eldest to bed at night, at a time she was also struggling with the arrival of her brother.

We bought our son a baby doll and a doll's bottle, so that he could feed his baby when I fed his sister. The novelty soon wore off, but I think it really helped for the first couple of weeks.

Bing was our saviour! Every time I had to breastfeed, we watched an episode of Bing. They're just long enough to last for a feed and keep a toddler's attention.

When the baby needs to nap

When your firstborn was a baby and needed to nap, it was easy to create an oasis of peace and quiet to enable the longest, easiest naps possible. Now, it can often feel as if you're trying to get your new baby to nap in the middle of the monkey enclosure at the zoo. I know well the frustration of having just managed to get the baby to sleep, only to have your toddler jump on top of the two of you/your preschooler singing Disney songs at the top of their lungs/your school-aged child rushing in with a life-or-death, need-to-tell-you-right-now piece of information. But second babies quickly become adept at snoozing in even the most raucous of environments, and this usually means that naps become easier as they grow because they tend to be infinitely more flexible sleep-wise than your firstborn.

This doesn't mean, however, that the early days and weeks are easy. They often aren't and can be incredibly frustrating. The following ideas can help, until the new baby becomes adjusted to loud and busy sleeping spaces:

- **Get out of the house!** Trying to keep your firstborn cooped up and creating a space that even vaguely resembles quiet for your newborn to nap in is asking for trouble. Get everyone wrapped up, if it's cold or, if it's sunny, grab the sunscreen and hats and get out. Go for a drive, if your baby is OK in the car; take the pram and go for a walk to the park in the hope the baby will sleep in the pram while your older child can let off steam playing; or take yourself out for a coffee. Being around other adults, even if you don't know them, can often provide a much-needed sanity check.

- **Use the sling.** I know my answer to most problems in the early days and weeks is to use a sling, but that's because they are so brilliant at making almost any situation easier. Pop the baby in the sling while you play with your firstborn or go for a walk: the baby gets movement and the sound of your heartbeat which provide comfort and your firstborn gets your free hands and the possibility of getting up and going somewhere or doing something.

- **Play some white noise.** White noise can really help newborns sleep. There are plenty of apps and downloads you can play (see Resources, p. 270). And the bonus is that not only does the white noise help to soothe the baby to sleep, but it also drowns out a lot of the noise the older child makes – a win–win scenario.

- **Go for a family nap.** Toddlers and preschoolers can be manic when they're overtired. Encouraging them to join you for a nap on the big bed with the baby in a co-sleeper crib or following bedsharing safety guidelines (see p. 270) can work well. The bonus here is that you can doze off too.

I asked some mothers how they coped when their babies needed to nap, but their firstborns had other ideas. Here's what they said:

> I used a sling a lot. I don't know how I would have coped without it. I pretty much kept my baby in a sling all day every day for the first six months. I quickly learned to breastfeed in it, leaving me available as much as possible for my older child, meaning I could meet the needs of both children.

> We used to go out for a car ride. The car had magical properties for both of my children, thankfully. I used to drive for twenty minutes to get them both to sleep, park up and read a book for half an hour while they napped, then drive home when one of them began to stir.

> My baby was born in the summer, so we had the fan on a lot. It was very noisy and used to really help the baby sleep; plus, it also muffled some of the noise from my older son!

> Go for a walk. That was my answer to everything. If the baby didn't sleep or the three-year-old was grouchy, we'd throw on our wellies and our jackets and get outside with the baby in the sling. My daughter was happy puddle-jumping and the baby used to go to sleep almost instantly in the sling.

What to do when they both cry at the same time

One of the hardest things about life in the early days with two children – and for months after that – is deciding what to do when both children cry at the same time. There is nothing so heart-wrenching as knowing both of your children need you, but only having one pair of hands and the ability to comfort one at a time. The realisation that you're going to have to leave one to cry is horrible. *Really* horrible – especially if you've never left your child to cry before.

The first time it happened to me, I panicked. My older son had fallen over and hurt himself and his crying had woken the baby who was crying because he was not ready to be awake and needed help to get back to sleep. I had a split second to try to decide who to prioritise. Often, people will prioritise the baby, because their cries are so piercing and emotive. You probably spent the whole of your firstborn's babyhood responding to their cries as quickly as possible. It feels wrong, therefore, to ignore the baby. However, sometimes, the older child really does need you more. In the example I gave, I comforted my older son first. He was in pain, his knee was bleeding and if I hadn't comforted him first, his crying would have continued to distress the baby. So I did what I could. I moved the baby in his basket close to my son and me on the sofa. My son sat on my lap as I dressed his knee and hugged him, and all the while I tried to jiggle the basket and 'sshh' my baby as best I could. By the time my oldest was quiet and calm again, the baby had fallen asleep. I felt absolutely wretched. I had allowed my baby to cry himself to sleep. It was not a parenting method I ever wanted to use. In this case though, I saw no other way. I had to leave one of them to cry and I had to decide who needed me most at the time. The baby was not in pain and I hoped that by speaking to him and trying to rock him, I had provided some comfort. I know if I had ignored my toddler, I would have felt a lot worse and, potentially, it would have caused more issues down the line, if he began to resent his brother for getting attention when he really needed me.

I don't think there is a right answer. If the baby was hurt, sick, overheating, too cold or hadn't fed in a long time, I probably would have prioritised him. I truly think that all you can do in this situation is to quickly triage needs in your head, take a deep breath and calm one child and then the other as soon as you can. Mostly though, you need to be kind to yourself. You can't do everything at once. Letting your baby or older child cry while you tend to their sibling, but trying all the while to provide comfort in whatever way you can, even if only verbally, is categorically not the same thing as allowing them to 'cry it out' to sleep train.

Try the following four steps when both children cry at the same time:

1. **Think about how you can prevent upset for the baby as much as possible.** With a newborn, I would be fully utilising a sling and carrying the baby as much as possible, all day if necessary. At this point, your newborn's needs are to be fed, to be clean, to be warm and to be held. The latter is totally fulfilled by the sling.

2. **Think about how you can prevent upsets for the toddler as much as possible.** First you need to understand that young children cry and tantrum – that's just what they do. That's not necessarily bad and it doesn't have to be stopped immediately. What you do need to do is to support your firstborn. Tell them that you are there for them, tell them that you understand how they feel and ask them if they would like a hug – one-handed if necessary. My focus at this point would be on the toddler as much as possible.

3. **Do some super-charged bonding.** When possible, I would spend some one-to-one time with each child, while the other is cared for by your partner, a friend or a relative. This time is all about cramming as much love and understanding in as possible with each child. Especially your firstborn.

4. **Accept your limitations and prioritise.** Realistically, it is unlikely you can tend to both children at the same time. Ask yourself whose need is the most pressing, and tend to that child first. The other child will cry and, unfortunately, this is something that will happen many, many times in the years to come. As soon as you can, scoop them up, empathise and apologise to them. Tell them that they are just as important to you as their sibling.

You also need to forgive yourself. It is hard and it can take time but you will do it. Then you will see the great bond that your children will form, and you will realise it was worth it and that they don't remember the times that they had to cry. It involves lots of work on your part: keeping your temper and 'time out' for you. The next chapter looks at ways in which you can stay calm amid the chaos if this is not something that comes easily to you, as it isn't for most mothers.

Getting out of the house with two

Getting out of the house with one baby seems like a mammoth task when you're a new parent. Getting out of the house with two children, when one of them is a newborn, often feels impossible. Pretty soon, I guarantee you will become highly skilled at getting everybody out, fully dressed and on time; in the interim though, don't rush yourself.

The military-style organisation of getting a growing family out of the door is a learned skill. I remember clearly the triumph of having finally got my toddler dressed and with his shoes on, only to discover that the baby needed his nappy changing just as we were about to leave. New nappy on and ready to go once again, I turned around to find a naked toddler. If it hadn't been so stressful, it would have been funny. Living the reality, however, it was hard to see the humour in it.

Before I had kids, I was always early wherever I went. When I had my firstborn, I struggled to just about make it to places on time. When I had my second, we were lucky if we arrived within thirty minutes of the agreed time. There are only two solutions here.

First, plan, plan and plan some more. Get things ready the night before. Pack what you think you'll need to take and then pack the same amount again. Have a back-up meeting time or plan, if the first doesn't work out. And plan online shopping well in advance of running out of any groceries, so that you only need to go out if you really need to.

The second solution is to accept your new normal – for a while that, is. Accept that the unexpected happens and you'll probably be late. Stop apologising and instead thank people for waiting for you. It's amazing what changing 'Sorry I'm late again' to 'Thanks so much for waiting for me' does to your confidence and self-esteem.

Some second-time mothers shared some of their secrets to getting out of the house. Here's what they said:

Preparing as much as possible the night before to make life easier for all is key and really helped me organise our lives. I purchased a set of five plastic drawers and use one per child, filling each week with clothes to make dressing a quicker process.

Use online grocery shopping. Start a few weeks before the baby comes, so you can find the shop that suits. It's been brilliant and definitely saves the stress of a toddler and baby, plus heavy trolley.

Get out of the house, but plan trips carefully. I went for enclosed spaces where my toddler couldn't escape if I was seeing to the baby e.g. friends' houses, gated parks and soft play.

Set your watch an hour fast. You'll soon forget that you did it and you might just make it to places on time!

Pack the car the night before with everything you'll need, so in the morning you'll just need to get the children ready.

Ask yourself if you really need to go to the baby class or soft play. Even if you planned it. Sometimes it stresses you far more because you're putting pressure on yourself. I found being flexible and not actually planning anything was key to my survival in the first couple of months.

Bedtime with two children

One of the questions I'm asked most frequently about life with a second baby and an older child, is how to do bedtime with two. There are two ways to answer this, depending on whether or not you are the only adult around at bedtime.

Bedtime with two adults present

If two adults are present, I strongly recommend that you don't have a combined, joint sibling bedtime, unless both children go to sleep easily and sleep 'well' all night – which, when you have a baby in the mix, is pretty unlikely!

In the early days, at least, I believe it is far better to keep bedtimes separate. When two adults are present at bedtime (and these don't necessarily have to be both the children's parents) each adult should focus on one child only, ideally swapping every night. Alternating caregivers works well for several reasons. Firstly, it allows both adults to form a good bond with the new baby, meaning the baby is more prone to take comfort from somebody other than Mum at night. Secondly, it means that your firstborn gets to spend bedtime with you three or four times per week, which is so important for bonding and reconnection, and which, in turn, impacts on their behaviour both in the daytime and at night. Finally, this flexibility means that both children should accept either adult putting them to bed in the future should one of you have to be away at night. If you have a baby who is breastfed, then I recommend that the other adult does all of the baby's bedtime routine on their 'baby night', right up to the final feeding to sleep, at which point the mother takes over the baby, while the other adult finishes settling the older child.

Here's a worked example with a baby and an older child, when it is a 'firstborn night' for the mother:

7 p.m.   Baby in the bath with Adult Two, while the mother reads the older child stories, plays quietly or chats in their bedroom or gives them a bedtime snack.

7.10 p.m. Baby and Adult Two go into the bedroom for a massage, while the older child is having a bath with the mother.

7.20 p.m. Mother and older child go into the bedroom where the older child will sleep, while Adult Two is getting the baby dressed in the bathroom.

7.30 p.m. Mother reads a bedtime story to the older child, gives them a hug, while Adult Two is with the baby (preferably in a different bedroom, if your home has two bedrooms or more; if not, quietly in the same bedroom).

7.35 p.m. Adult Two then stays with the older child, while the mother feeds the baby to sleep.

8 p.m. Hopefully, both children are asleep around this time. If the baby is asleep and the older child is still awake, the mother comes back to the child for hugs. Adult Two can then leave.

Bedtime with one adult present

This one is much harder. If at all possible, try to enlist help for an hour a day, at bedtime. If this is not practically or financially viable, my advice is to get through bedtime as best you can. This often means doing things you would not ordinarily do if there were two adults available, such as watching TV or playing with tablets or smartphones. This isn't ideal, but with a lack of alternatives it can be helpful. Just make sure that any devices are switched to 'night mode' to reduce the amount of blue light emitted, as it inhibits the release of melatonin, the sleep hormone.

There are three ways you can do things.

1. Oldest child asleep first

Here, you need to rely on something occupying the baby while you get their older sibling to sleep – a bouncy chair, playmat or sling, even in front of a screen (remember, I would do things here that aren't optimal if they keep the baby calm and entertained for longer). If you go down this route, it is vital that you get some one-to-one time in with your toddler when you do have adult help. Audiobooks and special children's relaxation recordings can be very useful here (you will find details in the Resources page 270), so that you can leave the older child sometimes when they are drowsy, or encourage them to close their eyes and listen, while you focus on the baby (in the same room).

2. Baby asleep first

Here, you need to rely on something occupying the older child. Screens usually come out tops again, especially if they are restricted at other times of the day. No, it's not ideal, but it is often the best alternative. A calm child who has been exposed to screens is better than a distressed one who wasn't. Again, remember to set screens to night mode to limit the effects of blue light exposure as much as possible. The proviso here is that you empathise with the child and let them know how much you really want to spend some time with them alone at bedtime when the baby is asleep, this encourages them to be quiet while you get the baby to sleep as quickly as possible, knowing that their time is coming.

3. Both asleep at the same time

This is the most common option if you are family bedsharing and tandem breastfeeding. But I have to say it's the one I would least recommend, simply as it is so hard to focus on both children at the same time and one may stop the other from sleeping. It seems like a wonderful idea and it works well for some families, but it can often result in long, drawn-out bedtimes. If it does work for you though, that's great – embrace it!

The early days with two children can be tricky, but you'll be surprised at how quickly you all adapt. The 'beautiful chaos' quickly becomes your new normal and life before four slowly starts to fade away, until you struggle to remember what it was like with only one child.

All families find their own groove – the things that work for them, whether that's related to getting out of the house, helping a baby to nap while entertaining an older child or tackling bedtime alone with two children. I've often thought that experience of parenting more than one child could make a fantastic addition to a CV: you become a pro at tackling crowd control, you develop military-grade organisational skills and have the ability to keep people happy, when they have different wants and needs – all of which would be welcomed in any workplace!

What you need to remember is that things do start to fall into place much quicker than you expect. Sometimes, however, a few niggly problems can remain, and that's what the next chapter will look at.

Chapter 10

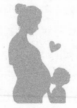

Difficult Reactions and Tricky Behaviours

Sometimes, despite the best preparation, and any excitement they may have felt about the arrival of a new sibling, children can really struggle with it when it happens. Difficult behaviours are not uncommon and often include violence directed towards the baby, parents or peers, sulking and withdrawal, shunning of your attention or the opposite – becoming incredibly clingy. Lapses in previously learned skills can also follow the arrival of the new baby, with toilet training, sleep (including bedtime resistance and increased night waking), eating and talking regressions topping the list. This chapter will look at these behaviours, understanding why they happen and, most importantly, how to reduce them and get your happy firstborn back again.

When do tricky behaviours most commonly arise?

There is a bit of a myth suggesting that tricky behaviours occur only as an immediate reaction to the arrival of a new sibling. I'm often contacted by struggling second-time parents who say to me, 'Well, it can't be the baby any more because he's nine months old now!' Many parents think that because the second baby is no longer a newborn, the time for any difficult reactions has long passed. This really isn't the case. Some children can react instantly to the arrival of a new baby, others, though, take things in their stride for the first few weeks and even months, only to react much further down the line. The timing of the reaction obviously depends on individual children and family circumstances, but I tend to find that the reactions in the very early days happen because of immediate shock and upheaval, whereas those that happen further down the line tend to occur once the older child has realised the baby is here to stay and goes off the idea of having a sibling. Often, this is when the baby becomes mobile and starts to touch the older child's toys, or when parents begin to share bedtime routines once the baby is no longer a delicate newborn. I believe that almost any behaviours children show within the first year of having a new sibling can be chalked up to the arrival of the baby, whether they happen one week or eleven months later.

The other point I should add here is that not all children respond negatively to the arrival of a new sibling. Some will adjust easily and love every moment of being a new big brother or sister. So I don't want to scare you into thinking that you are on borrowed time if you currently have a perfectly behaved older child. Yes, it is more likely that families will experience tricky behaviours and reactions, but absolutely not all do. I hope you are one of the lucky ones!

Memories of becoming an older sibling

Before we look at the most common tricky behaviours that manifest when new babies arrive in the family, I'd like to spend some time thinking about *why* they might happen. If you have a younger sibling, do you remember how you felt after they arrived?

I often think the best answers to parenting dilemmas can be solved when we think back to our own childhoods and consider how we felt when we misbehaved, and what we really needed from our parents at the time. I asked some adults how they felt when a younger sibling arrived. This is what they told me:

There's about two and half year's difference between my sister and me. I remember going to visit her in the hospital and everyone coming to our house to see my sister. I was sat quietly on the side while they were giving my little sister gifts. I honestly did not understand why, suddenly, they didn't even want to hold me! I've been told that when she was born I used take her bottle and start drinking it, take her nappy off and try to put it on or just try to destroy her toys. I didn't know what was going on. The health visitor said I was 'trouble' and put me in a playgroup. English wasn't my first language at that point and I remember soiling myself, not knowing how to ask to go to the toilet. After that point, I just remember not wanting much to do with my sister – and to this day, our relationship hasn't been the best. I now have a twenty-month-old daughter. If we have a second baby, I am going to do everything in my power to make her feel included and be part of the family. I would never want her to feel like she had to compete for attention.

I remember being disappointed that I had another brother and not a sister. I also think having a younger baby brother triggered off my biting phase, as I did not know or understand how I felt about him being around.

I remember feeling really upset because my mum always seemed to be holding the baby and didn't give me as many cuddles as she had before. I guess in my three-year-old head I felt that the lack of cuddles meant she loved me less than the new baby.

Jealousy towards the new baby

There is no denying that the main reason for tricky behaviour after the arrival of a younger sibling is jealousy. Having said that, I hate the term jealousy when used in this scenario, because I think it completely undermines what the child is feeling. Jealousy is an unpleasant and undesirable trait. To say that a child is jealous implies that they are not very nice, and that their jealousy is something they could control, if they wanted to. Describing the older sibling's feelings in this way predisposes parents towards punishing them in some way for those feelings.

A much better word to describe the swirl of big and difficult emotions that new siblings feel is grief. This helps us to understand the loss that the child is feeling – the loss of the family that once was, the loss of your full attention towards them, the loss of their belief that you would always be there for them when they needed you and the loss of their place in the family as 'the baby'. The word grief succeeds where the word jealousy fails, in allowing us to see that children aren't being deliberately naughty or selfish. Grief helps us to empathise, support and react with compassion, rather than anger, punishment and annoyance. So my top tip to help both you and your child through the transition is to drop all talk of jealousy from your vocabulary and switch to the word grief instead. Viewing your child as grieving will ensure that your reaction and response towards them are always in their best interests and will be far, far more effective.

I spoke to some parents about their children's reactions when their new baby sibling arrived. As you read through their responses, replace the words jealous and jealousy with grief and grieving and observe how differently you feel about the children in these scenarios.

My daughter was so jealous of her baby brother. She would be very rough with him and get between him and me. I found this really distressing, as one of the main reasons my husband and I decided to have a second child was so our daughter would have a sibling, as we are both close to our own respective siblings. My daughter is incredibly jealous and almost possessive of me. For example, she might be playing nicely on one side of the room, and out of the corner of her eye she will see my son sitting on my lap. She will immediately come over and state that it's her turn on my lap and push him off. I constantly worry that my son will feel his sister doesn't care about him or that I give her more attention because she demands it. I think she would be a different kid if she had been older when he was born.

My eldest son remembers his sister coming home from hospital. He was three years old at the time. He tells me that he liked her at first but didn't understand that she was staying for good! He said when he realised that she'd be staying, he was jealous.

My son was incredibly jealous after his sister arrived. He had previously been a happy-go-lucky, easy and mild-mannered little boy, yet suddenly, he started to yell, refuse to do what he was told and even started to be violent towards us on occasion. The jealousy was at its worse in the early weeks, but even a year on, he's still prone to bouts of jealousy.

My daughter was really excited about her new baby sister arriving, until she arrived, that is! My goodness, I had no idea she would be so jealous. She's normally great at sharing with her cousins, so I didn't expect any problems with the baby. She would frequently scream when I was feeding her sister and hated me cuddling the baby too much. I really struggled with her jealousy. It was so out of character for her.

When the new baby was born my son was so jealous. Things got really bad when the baby was three weeks old and he bit her. I went to get us some lunch in the kitchen and left my daughter in the crib and my son watching a TV programme. I was gone for two or three minutes at most. When I came back into the room I found a big red mark on my daughter's arm, but my son refused to admit it was him. Obviously, it was, and I know he did it because he was jealous of her, as previously that morning he had told me that he wanted her to live somewhere else.

How did changing the word jealous to grief change how you felt about the children in these stories? Did it help you to empathise with them more? Did it make you view them more positively? Did it help you to understand how best to deal with their behaviour? The way we respond to grief is very different to the way we respond to jealousy. This is a point I'd like you to keep in mind as we work through this chapter.

Hurting the baby – or you

Acting violently towards either yourself, or the baby and sometimes peers, day-care staff and other adults is a common reaction to a new baby arriving. Underneath all these behaviours lie two emotions: grief and frustration.

Violent reactions towards new siblings are most commonly seen in children who are not yet verbal or who have difficulty expressing themselves – particularly their emotions – through words. The feelings build up inside, and without an adequate way to release them, or to express themselves, violence is often the way that the overwhelming feelings spill out.

Violence towards the baby is an obvious reaction to the thing that has brought about all the pain the child is feeling, just as we, as adults, may be tempted to lash out physically at a loved one who has deeply upset us. The difference here is that as adults, we can control our impulses, as well as verbalise them if we so choose. Children can do neither of these things. The violence is a simple outpouring of painful emotions.

The same is true of violence towards parents – the people the child thought they could trust, but who have brought this new baby into their lives. Violence towards peers, day-care staff and other carers is just another expression of frustration and grief, and it is often triggered by something completely unrelated to the baby – for instance, being asked to tidy up or share a toy.

Parents can find violence incredibly hard to deal with. Aside from the obvious worry about the new baby being hurt, it can be very hard to not take it personally and be anxious about what you did to create such a menace. Friends, family and health professionals may advise parents to ignore the bad behaviour, punish their child for hurting or praise and reward them every time they are good. However, these common discipline methods only serve to make the child feel worse. If you want the child to behave better – and to stop the violence – the answer is simple: you must make them feel better (see p. 229 for more on this).

Being over-attentive to their sibling

At the opposite end of the scale to violence is the new big brother or sister who will not leave the baby alone. They can often be overzealous in their affection, deliberately waking the baby up, being rough with their cuddles and a little too overenthusiastic with their kisses and caresses. But all these behaviours are underlined with a very positive emotion indeed – love. In time, your child will become naturally less enthusiastic, as the excitement and novelty of the baby fade. Until that happens, make sure that you teach your child how to handle their new sibling and put some strict boundaries in place; for instance, they should never pick the baby up if you are not in the room and they should never wake the baby up if they are sleeping. If your firstborn is a little too young to understand, then the simple answer here is to never leave them alone together. And if you must leave the room to do something, even if it's going to the toilet, then carry the baby with you in a sling.

Indifference towards the baby

Sometimes I think one of the hardest behaviours for parents to cope with when a second baby is born is the sheer indifference that children commonly show towards their new sibling.

I speak to so many parents who say, 'I don't know what I was expecting, but I was expecting something! She doesn't seem to love the baby, but she doesn't hate the baby either. There's just nothing.' The biggest problem here is the difference between what you usually imagine and what really happens.

Babies are cute, but they're pretty boring. They don't make good playmates, and toddlers, preschoolers and even older children quickly lose interest. Playing together doesn't tend to happen until much later, towards the end of the first year of the baby's life or even later. So indifference towards their new sibling in the first few months is common and entirely natural for children. The lack of interest and bonding doesn't mean it will never happen. It's just likely to take longer than you imagined. The best advice I can give here is to be patient and trust that it will come naturally in time. You don't need to encourage or force it. You just need to wait.

Reactions towards parents

It is very common after the birth of a second baby for the firstborn child to act strangely towards their parents, usually their mother. These reactions, once again, stem from grief (see page 217) and confusion – confusion as to their new place in your affection and confusion surrounding your decision to introduce a new baby into the family. I always imagine that children can feel as if their parents are in some way trying to replace them by having another baby, or perhaps they feel that they are not good enough for their parents. Either way, the baby can often make them feel insecure with regard to their place in their parents' world – particularly the parent who carried and birthed the baby: the mother.

The two most common reactions I see are shunning affection and deliberately avoiding kisses and hugs from the mother, and being clingy, desperate to be with her as much as possible. Both of these behaviours are saying the same thing: 'Do you love me as much as you used to? I feel unsure of your love.'

Both clinginess and indifference can be incredibly hard for mothers to cope with. The thing to do here is to stay calm, not blame yourself or take your child's reaction too personally. They're not the first child to react this way and they won't be the last. The best that you can do is to keep reassuring them of your love and be patient. Avoid punishment, exclusion, separation and rewards; these all aim to hurry the resolution of the child's uncomfortable feelings, but often make them far, far worse.

Destructive behaviour

Children can often exhibit destructive behaviour towards objects, as well as people, after the birth of a new sibling. Throwing, kicking and shoving objects are common, as is destroying favourite toys or presents, especially those given to the new baby. Grief is the ultimate underlying emotion here once again (see p. 217), along with a good dose of frustration.

Destructive behaviour in children is a classic sign of externalising emotions – that is, releasing emotions that are too uncomfortable for them to hold onto, in much the same way as when we are angry and feel like punching the wall or ripping something up. Once again, the difference is that as adults, we have fully developed brains and can self-regulate our emotions. By that, I mean that we can breathe deeply and control our anger and, ultimately, we can calm ourselves again without the need to destroy anything. Children don't have this level of sophisticated cognitive thought. So instead of working to dial down their emotions internally, they explode and let them out externally, like a boiling pot without a lid, spilling everywhere.

This isn't 'naughty' behaviour; not deliberately, anyway. It's a sign of a child who is struggling with the big feelings that come with becoming a new big brother or sister and all the expectations and challenges that their new role brings. Of course, it's not OK that they go on a path of destruction. You need to calmly and firmly say, 'Stop! I will not let you destroy that!' and take away the endangered object. But after that, you need to treat them with compassion and help them to release their feelings in a safe and supported manner. Punishing, ignoring and excluding may train a child to not destroy things, but it does nothing to safely defuse the ticking emotional bomb that is causing the behaviour. To stop the destruction, you need to deal with the root cause – the grief and the frustration – and ways to do this are explained on pages 229–231.

This mum talks about her daughter's violent reaction to the new baby, and what helped:

> My daughter demonstrated the most extreme and volatile mood swings. We had never seen anything like it. Huge tantrums over seemingly random things. So many tears and screaming. We just rode it out mostly and tried to understand. We think that she was demonstrating control where she could because she felt out of control. So we just tried to acknowledge and understand her feelings. Of course, there have been soooo many times we have lost it, or just acknowledged nicely through gritted teeth because to be honest, this shiz has been bloody hard work and continues to be so. She wakes the baby up when I have had no sleep and have only just got him back to sleep . . . argh! It's all still the steepest knife-edge learning curve. Sometimes you just don't have the energy to understand that a child screaming at you because you gave them a pink plate instead of a green one is actually telling you that they need attention and are worried about being a big sister.

Regression

Regressing behaviour is very common among children who have just become a new big brother or sister, and the three main areas that it occurs in are eating, potty training and sleep. This is no coincidence – because a child who is feeling that the rest of their life is out of control will tend to seek control in those areas where they have autonomy.

The other cause of regressing behaviour is the desire to want to be little again: little gets affection, little gets love, little gets attention. And these are all the things that the now big sibling feels that they lack. So if babies get all the attention now, then surely acting like one is a good way to recover whatever they feel they have lost. Firstborns can often start talking in baby speak, with a high-pitched voice and babbling sounds; they may decide they want to suck a dummy again or be covered by a baby blanket; and they may be drawn to the baby toys. Go with it. Allow them to be little again if that's what they want. The behaviour will wane naturally.

Eating regressions

When new babies arrive, it is not uncommon for firstborns to see their baby brother or sister being cradled while breastfed or being given a bottle and to miss that closeness. Wanting to breast- or bottle-feed again is their attempt at recreating the bond of babyhood. Is there a problem with letting them do either? I really don't think so.

Children seem to forget how to breastfeed remarkably quickly after weaning, so usually after a few attempts to feed they will give up and accept that it is no longer for them. And the same applies to a bottle. (If they do want to try a bottle,

I would suggest giving them the slowest possible teat, so that they quickly get fed up with the slow flow of the milk.) Meeting their need in this instance is far easier than fighting it. The worst that could happen is that they have a bottle again temporarily, or perhaps breastfeed a little – neither of which is really a bad outcome at all, especially if they reduce any other tricky behaviour and make your life easier as a result.

Potty-training regressions

Potty training regressions can occur around the arrival of a new sibling for three reasons.

The first is that the emotional upset takes the child's focus away from controlling their bowel and bladder. If they have not been trained for long (and by that, I mean under a year), it's common to have accidents. When these happen, they need lots of reassurance and a reminder that it's OK.

The second reason is the same as the desire to breast- or bottle-feed again. They see the new baby wearing a nappy and equate nappy wearing with 'littleness' and being given lots of affection and attention. Asking to wear a nappy again can often be a sign of a child saying, 'I'm cute too. Please see me – I'm still little, even though I may seem big to you now!'

Finally, potty accidents can sometimes, but rarely, be deliberate. By that, I mean the child may choose to urinate or defecate in inappropriate places as a way to get attention. The answer here isn't to admonish them. Clear them up, but pay little attention to them; and there is certainly no need to put the child back in nappies or retrain them. The problem really has nothing to do with potty training at all. It is a cry for attention. Meet that need and the child will have no need to deliberately soil.

Recurrence of night waking and bedtime resistance

Sleep regressions are very, very common in firstborns after the arrival of a new baby. Sleep is so linked to our emotions, even in adulthood. As adults, if we're stressed, anxious, nervous or worried about something, then we'll struggle to sleep. It is no different for children, but often, it's worse – the emotional turmoil many face as a new sibling is seen clearly in their disrupted sleep. As adults, we can regulate some of those difficult emotions, rationalising them and finding practical ways to drift off to sleep – a meditation app, a mindfulness recording, some deep breathing. Young children can do none of these things.

The answer here is empathy, understanding and patience. Support the child through the emotions and their sleep will naturally improve. The worst thing you can do is try to implement sleep training, drop naps, mess around with bedtime, switch bedrooms or carry out any other change. Because change, ultimately, means more disruption and more tricky feelings. Keep everything the same, reassure and ride it out.

Bedtime resistance is also common among new big siblings. And this one is so obvious: they don't want to go to bed and be away from you, especially knowing that the baby will be with you all night. The previous chapter looked at other adults, especially partners, taking over bedtime with the older child every night, while Mum stays with the baby in the evening. This is completely the wrong thing to do from the firstborn's point of view. Mum should do bedtime for the eldest child as much as possible, while the partner is with the baby in another room. You could alternate, as per the example in the previous chapter, or, in an ideal world, you would be able to do bedtime with your eldest every night while your partner has the baby. This sounds counterintuitive, especially if you're breastfeeding. There is no easy way around this, aside from breastfeeding your baby just before your older child's bedtime, passing them over, leaving the room quickly and closing the door behind you, safe in the knowledge that they have just been fed and they are in the safe care of somebody who loves them. Even if they cry, it's not the same as them crying alone. So long as they are being held and offered comfort, the impact on their brain is nothing like it would be if they were crying alone. If your baby is happy in the sling, car or pram, it can be helpful if they can be taken out for a walk or a quick drive. This has a double benefit: it usually stops the tears much more easily than staying at home; and, secondly, if your baby does cry, you and your older child won't be as upset by it, as you won't hear them. This sounds incredibly harsh. Sadly, there is no getting away from crying when you have two children. You just need to keep reminding yourself that crying is OK so long as the baby is fully supported.

This special alone time at bedtime is the key to solving sleep dilemmas, whether that's night waking or bedtime resistance. It's also the key to all other behaviour dilemmas relating to the arrival of a new baby. Bedtime is a predictable constant. Throughout the day, you can remind your child, 'we'll have a huge hug at bedtime', if they're struggling and you need to be with the baby. Bedtime is like a little snippet of that time you shared together pre-baby. It allows you to snatch a few moments alone with your firstborn and, most importantly, it fulfils their need to have you all to themselves, if only for half an hour each day.

If you do not have a partner, or your partner is not at home at bedtime, then finding time to reconnect, one to one, with your eldest at other times is incredibly important. Perhaps you have other family members who could watch your baby for an hour or two once every couple of weeks, or a close friend who may be willing to do a babysitting swap with you. Reconnecting with your firstborn, without their sibling around, is ultimately the best way to reduce any difficult behaviour that they may be displaying as a result of feeling a lack of connection with you.

The five-step plan to resolving baby-related behaviour issues

The solution to all behaviour problems that arise in the wake of the arrival of a new baby in the family is time. Until that time passes, however, the following five steps can really help to reassure your child, which will eventually reduce their grief, frustration, confusion and, hopefully, their tricky behaviour.

1. **Show more understanding and empathy.** Remind yourself that your child is not jealous or being deliberately malicious; they are grieving, and they are hurting. Their behaviour shows they are struggling and they need your help. Remember – difficult reactions can happen months after the baby's arrival too. When you empathise with your child's feelings, the way that you behave with them is naturally different. You are likely to be calmer and more patient towards them, and they will pick up on that.

2. **Recognise their feelings.** Acknowledging your child's feelings and showing them that you understand how they feel can go a long way to resolving their behaviour. By saying things like, 'It's so hard sometimes when the baby needs to feed so much, isn't it? I miss our hugs; I bet you do too?' you are recognising your child's feelings without them needing to verbalise them. This shows your child that you get it. You get them. And you're on the same team.

3. **Keep the lines of communication open.** Encouraging your child to communicate their feelings with you in whatever way they can is very helpful. If they are older, then instigate conversations with them about their feelings; bedtime is a great time for this. If they are pre-verbal, then teaching some simple sign language can help to remove frustration. And if they are verbal, but are struggling to understand emotions, then try reading books explaining them, so that they can point out pictures or characters they feel are like them.

4. **Maintain a close connection.** Connection is the key. Your child is mourning the relationship you once had and feeling pushed out by the new arrival. You need to appreciate what a huge deal this is to them and help them to feel connected with you again. Doing bedtime, without the baby, every, or every other, night is a great first step. But children can need more: an hour in the park together every Saturday morning, while the baby stays home with another adult or swimming together, without the baby every Sunday afternoon – something predictable that occurs every week is the ideal. Once the baby is older, or you feel able to leave them for several hours at a time, then planning some special Mum-and-son/daughter time is important. Ideally, a whole day or, if not, a whole morning or afternoon together, just enjoying each other's company, doing something fun together, while somebody else takes care of the baby, can work miracles. This special day/time should be as well as, not instead of, the more frequent bedtimes and short park visits.

5. **Be patient and persistent.** Unfortunately, none of these techniques will work quickly. They require perseverance, patience and persistence. Think in months. Having a

new sibling is a big deal, and it takes adjustment. Often, you will find certain behaviours recur further down the line, even after a period of relative calm. This is normal and, once again, they will pass. Eventually. In the meantime, the most important part of the puzzle is you. How you cope and react underpins everything.

Keeping calm and controlling your own behaviour

Parenting is undoubtedly the hardest job you will ever do. It is unrelenting. There is no sick pay, no duvet days when you're ill, no holiday pay, no 'away days', no personnel support or workplace counselling. It is an amazing, but often tortuous blend of constant physical and mental effort. Parenting one child is hard. Parenting two can often feel impossible.

For the first few years of parenting, I gave it my all and then some. Not only did I try to be all that I could for my kids, I also tried to be the perfect homemaker, the perfect cook, the perfect event planner, the perfect friend and the perfect wife. Clearly, this was totally unsustainable. I became exhausted, frequently sick with colds and other viruses. I lost a lot of 'me' in those early years. And my inability to see that I needed nurturing just as much as my children meant that I became short-tempered, I 'lost it' at my kids more than I would care to admit and, although I loved raising them, I began to resent them too. This drove a wedge in our connection and, combined with my lack of patience and spiralling self-control, we entered a dark period. I became 'shouty mum' – so far from the mum I aspired to be.

There was no one defining moment that made me 'see the light'. It was a gradual realisation that I couldn't go on as I was. I wasn't being the parent I wanted to be, and I could see the negative reflection of this in the behaviour of my children, especially my firstborn. Something had to change – and for the first time, I realised that it was me.

I finally understood that in my quest to be 'all-present' for my children, I had neglected myself, and that was the worst thing I could have done. My children both needed a calm, patient mum, not the angry, stressed one I had become. I realised that, for their sake, I needed to take better care of myself.

Self-care can often feel like an ominous task, but I think that's mostly because we misunderstand it. There are three widespread myths that I hear again and again about self-care:

1. **It takes too much time.** Self-care can seem like yet another thing added to your ever-growing 'to-do list'. You probably feel like you don't have the time or energy for it, but I can tell you now that if you don't find time for yourself, you're going to have to find the time to deal with difficult behaviour from your children, not just now, but in the years to come. Either way, you're going to have to make the time and energy to deal with it, so you can either prevent it or deal with the aftermath. And the beauty of self-care is that it really doesn't have to take much time. It can be slotted into your daily routine, even with a toddler and a baby, because on the simplest of levels it just means being more mindful of your own needs and feelings. You can do that while feeding a baby or changing a nappy. Awareness doesn't take time.

2. **It costs too much money.** Self-care can be totally free. Too many people think self-care means paying for a massage or joining a yoga class. It really doesn't. Yes, some people may incorporate these things into their self-care routine (I choose to go to a weekly Pilates class and have reflexology once a month), but, these things aren't

necessary. Self-care is a mindset; the big work goes on in your own head and that doesn't cost anything. Neither does sitting on your sofa and focusing on nothing but your breath for two minutes or telling yourself that 'I matter too'. Financial pressures are not a reason to not be kind to yourself.

3. **It means you have to be away from your children.** For some mothers, getting some time away from their children is vital. They need the breathing space, and if this is you, I can't recommend more strongly that you try to find a way to make it work – even for an hour a week. Others can't bear the thought of being away from their children, especially the baby, and doing so would make them more stressed. If that's you, it's perfectly possible to be more mindful towards your own needs with a baby at your breast and a toddler on your knee, if that's what you want. The beauty is, this is all about you, nobody else. How *you* feel is the only important aspect in self-care.

Implementing self-care

There are six important steps to self-care for mothers:

1. Start by accepting that your thoughts and feelings have a huge impact on your parenting. You are the key. You can't change how your children behave, if you don't first change how you feel. If you're stressed, anxious and angry then your children will be stressed, anxious and angry.

2. Acknowledge that it is not selfish to have your own needs and to fulfil them. You are the backbone of your family. You are in constant use. You get your car regularly serviced and your boiler checked each year. Why don't

you give yourself the same courtesy? If your car broke down with your children in it after years of neglect, you wouldn't blame the car – you would understand it was your fault for not taking care of it. The same goes for you too.

3. Take some time to think about what it is you need most. Is it time away from the children? Some peace and quiet to think? A way to offload? Some more sleep? Better food? More socialising with friends? Fewer playgroups and baby or toddler activities? Simplifying your life a little? Consider writing a list of what you need in your diary – a little like a self-care Christmas wish-list. I always feel that once something is written down, it becomes more serious.

4. Think about the simplest ways you can meet your needs and start with those. Maybe a bath to yourself with the door closed; reading a new novel instead of a parenting book; calling an old friend and talking about the past, or how tricky life with two children is (it always helps to feel that you're not alone); watching a cheesy romance instead of doing the washing.

5. Be kind to yourself daily and, most importantly, be forgiving. Start trying to be as nice to yourself as you are to everyone else.

6. Keep it going. While you may need an 'emergency self-care top-up' every now and again, this new way of thinking needs to become a permanent fixture. You can't dabble in self-care for a few days or weeks and then go back to neglecting your own needs. It's about having a new awareness that is constantly present in your life. Ultimately, this is the only way to control your temper and give your children the calm parent that they deserve. You're doing it for them – as much as, if not more than, for yourself.

These mums talked about how they coped on the tough days:

> The early days were hard, but you must remember the days are long, but the years are short; I used to say this to myself all the time while I sat on the floor cuddling my toddler who was having a tantrum and feeding my baby. I see parents now struggling and always go have a quiet word saying, "Well done, you're doing a great job". It is tough, and people worry that others may judge if they see their child having a tantrum, but it is all normal.

> I realised quickly that I couldn't be everything to both children, especially if I didn't look after myself. So I made time for myself once a week to go to my old yoga class. It really helped so much being away from the children for an hour a week, just catching time to breathe and relax. I was definitely a better mum for it when I came back after a class.

> I used to close my eyes and picture us all in ten or twenty years' time, sitting together as a family, with the girls as good friends. That picture kept me going on many a tough day.

> I think knowing that I wasn't alone really helped. Speaking to other second-time mums and hearing that they were struggling made me feel much better. I felt a bit useless before. I thought everybody was coping but me. Realising I was normal was a huge help. I felt like I could breathe again.

I'd like to end this chapter with Holly's story. Holly talks about the importance of self-care and sharing the load, as well as spending quality time connecting with her firstborn and communicating about their emotions well.

Holly's story

My biggest tip to any new second-time mother is not to try doing it all yourself. Sharing the housework with my husband and both of us spending time with the children – we either have one child each or one of us will have both while the other does chores, etc. – is so important. I try to spend as much time as possible with my eldest. When we take care of one each, I tend to do more of the caring for our youngest, and my husband our eldest. This is mostly for practical reasons. However, where possible, I try to spend quality time with our eldest, which also gives my husband a chance to get to know our youngest more. I also find that getting my eldest daughter involved in the care of her little brother works well. She loves this and will happily do useful things, such as bring nappies, or entertain him while I am doing something else, such as showering or cooking. This will always be within a short distance of me, so that I can see them, but it is a really big help and has also allowed them to bond more.

I also really recommend talking to your eldest about what is happening. I found this a helpful way of acknowledging and validating both her and our feelings about all the changes that were happening. When my eldest pushes boundaries, or engages in somewhat destructive behaviour, it helps to take a few deep breaths and ask if she wants a hug. The answer is almost always yes, and this tends to defuse the situation almost immediately. I also make sure that I apologise to her when I get it wrong or cannot be there in ways that I could before.

I really try to make as much time to spend one-to-one with my firstborn as possible, or to focus on a bit of self-care. For instance, making the most of the baby's many naps to either spend time with his sister or do something nice for me. I have also continued with the childcare arrangements we already had for our eldest, with a nanny taking care of her for three days per week. This means I can spend some time alone with the baby as well and have some much-needed downtime. Our daughter loves her nanny, which helps!

Most importantly, utilise and mobilise as much help and support as possible. We don't have any family in this country, so have got a nanny that we 'share' with another family. This means childcare costs are the same as a nursery, but it gives us a lot more flexibility. On days when things don't go to plan, it doesn't matter if we are still in our pyjamas when she arrives. I also focus on going to bed early. I now go to bed around eight-thirty, as this ensures I get between six and eight (broken) hours of sleep. Any less and I don't cope as well. My husband stays up after we've all gone to bed and cleans the kitchen and tidies up, as he then gets to sleep for six to seven hours without waking up. Once or twice a week, my husband and I try to spend at least thirty minutes catching up with each other properly and talking a bit about what is going on in our lives. When we don't, we can easily start having mis-understandings and getting a bit annoyed with each other.

Finally, my top tip is to accept that this is how it will be for a while now and try to focus on the positives when things feel hard. We've made a lot of sacrifices, in terms of our own interests and social lives, but we still try to maintain elements of these where possible. Seeing the children happy and knowing we are giving them the best start in life we can is very rewarding though. There will be more time for other things when the children are a bit older.

It can often feel that you are alone with your struggles after a second baby arrives. You can find yourself questioning if there is something wrong with you, or with your child. There really isn't though. Whatever you experience after your second baby is born, I can assure you, as I've said, that you are not alone. Tricky transitions and difficult behaviours are common after welcoming a second baby into your family. It doesn't mean you've done anything wrong. It doesn't mean you've prepared your firstborn insufficiently and it doesn't mean that you're not a great parent. What your child needs is for you to see them for the 'baby' they once were, and sometimes still need to be. They need to feel reassured that your love for them has not changed, they need to reconnect and they need to be supported through any grief and frustration. The only way that you can do this effectively is to take care of yourself. Self-sacrifice only results in exhaustion. To take care of your firstborn, you must start with taking care of yourself.

Chapter 11

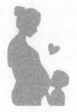

Sibling Love and Sibling Rivalry

I f you are like me, one of the top reasons that you had a second baby, was to provide your firstborn with a friend for life. As an only child, I can see the huge value in the gift of a sibling. In fact, I think it can be one of the most selfless things a parent can do for their child, despite the deep feelings of guilt and selfishness many parents feel in the immediate aftermath of the arrival of the new baby. Knowing that when you leave this earth, your child will not be alone, but instead have a family member they can rely on is peace of mind indeed. The trouble is, we put an awful lot of pressure on our children to be friends and an awful lot of blame on them, and ourselves, when they are not. But relationships, particularly familial ones, aren't perfect. Despite the Waltonsesque picture we may hold in our minds, real-life sibling relationships are often fraught with bickering, as evidenced by the fact that an internet search for the term 'sibling rivalry' returns over 5 million results.

I don't believe it is possible to have two or more children and not have any sibling rivalry, and I think books and articles that promise to remove or stop it are unrealistic. I also happen to believe that sibling rivalry is not such a bad thing. This chapter will view sibling rivalry through a realistic lens – looking at why it happens, why it's entirely normal and why you shouldn't worry about it. It will also look at ways to take the edge off the sibling fights when they do happen and to reduce some of the stress over the coming years and, most importantly, how to raise children who will be there for each other in the years when perhaps you're no longer around – hopefully, in the distant future.

Why sibling rivalry can be a good thing

With so many resources giving parents advice to stop sibling fighting, we lose sight of the positive side of these seemingly negative interactions. Parents can be so eager to stop any fighting that they don't realise that most sibling fights provide wonderful communication education, personal growth and emotional literacy to both children. To aim to stop any sibling squabbles is not only naïve (because no family has siblings that don't fight!), but a lost learning opportunity for the children. So rather than getting stressed worrying about fighting siblings, my best advice is to accept the behaviour for the normal, common and positive thing that it is.

Research from Cambridge University has found that fighting siblings help each other's emotional development.[1] This is largely because the relationships help siblings to explore a wide variety of feelings in relation to social interaction, which can help them in future social situations, particularly when verbalising their feelings. Siblings who squabbled tended to have a more mature range and understanding of emotionally rich language, than those without siblings. The lead study researcher, Dr Claire Hughes, said that 'the balance of our evidence suggests that children's social understanding may be accelerated by their interaction with siblings in many cases. One of the key reasons for this seems to be that a sibling is a natural ally. They are often on the same wavelength, and they will tend to engage in the sort of pretend play that helps children to develop an awareness of mental states.'

In short, sibling fighting allows children to grow up practising social skills that will be necessary to see them peacefully through life. They get to practise the less positive side of relationships, tackle personal conflict and understand how their behaviour affects others in the safety of their own home, so that when they leave it, they carry with them the important lessons to future relationships. With no (or little) fighting, they lose the opportunity for this important emotional development. For parents, sibling rivalry can often be hard to handle and something that most seek to avoid (unsuccessfully), but for the children, it's a gift.

What to do when they fight

Despite the positives of sibling fighting, there is no denying that it is sometimes better for you to step in and intervene. The key here is in trying to strike a balance – one that allows the children to solve their own problems and work on their relationship, but stops them from seriously hurting each other. Stepping in and taking over generally doesn't help. It prevents children from learning how to resolve conflict without adult help, it disempowers them and it makes them less likely to try to resolve problems next time – which, ultimately, means more fights. Only get involved when somebody is getting hurt and the fighting is not abating, objects are being broken or the fighting does not seem to be resolving, after you've given the children plenty of time to sort out the problem themselves. Instead, sit tight for as long as you can. I aim to interfere in under a fifth of my children's fights, or even less if possible.

If you do need to intervene, the biggest point to be mindful of is that your role should be that of a mediator or a go-between, not a referee or judge – encouraging communication and self-resolution between both children, rather than taking over and providing a verdict. Here's what this might look like in practice – for this example, let's imagine the children are fighting over a toy that they both want; you have resisted intervening for ten minutes with no apparent signs of resolution:

You: What's happening here? I can hear two very angry and upset children.

Child A: I want the toy; she won't let me have it. I had it first.

Child B: That's not true. I had it first. I want it. He took it from me.

You: OK, it sounds like both of you are pretty upset. Can you think of a way to resolve this?

Child A: She should give me the toy and go away.

Child B: He gives me the toy back. It was mine first.

You: Hmmm, it would be great if I could magic another toy, so you could both have one. I'm not so sure your ideas would work because it means one of you would always be unhappy. Can you think of a way to resolve this where you're both happy?

Child A: I could have the toy now and she can have it tomorrow.

Child B: No, I should have it today and he can have it tomorrow.

You: I like the idea of sharing the toy, but tomorrow is quite a long time to wait if you both want to play with it now. Can you think of anything a bit better?

Child A: She can play with it after lunch.

Child B: No, you can play with it after lunch.

You: That sounds a bit better. But how do we decide who has it now? It seems that whoever doesn't get it now will be sad.

Child A: Maybe we could flip a coin?

Child B: We could play Rock, Paper, Scissors?

You: I don't have a coin on me, so we can't do that right now. But you could do Rock, Paper, Scissors. Is that OK, A?

Child A: I guess.

You: OK, let's go – one, two, three, Rock, Paper, Scissors. [Child B wins.]

Child A: That sucks.

Child B: Yay, it's mine!

You: A, I understand it sucks when you don't win, but remember, you get it after lunch. B, just remember, that after lunch it's your brother's for the rest of the day, OK?

Child B: OK.

You: Is that OK, A?

Child A: OK.

In this example, A and B reached a resolution together. Because they came up with the ideas, they have ownership and are more likely to accept the outcome. Talking through what was happening allowed both children to feel validated and heard by you and encouraged them to talk about how they were feeling. In time, this approach will help the children to understand and appreciate their sibling's feelings and eventually, they will complete this sort of process without your help. But it's important to be realistic. It's unlikely that children will reach this sort of mature resolution independently until they approach their teenage years, and even then, there will be many times when they revert back to the sort of behaviour they displayed as toddlers. Sibling-resolution techniques do help, but it takes years and years of practice before children utilise them automatically when they fight. This doesn't mean that your attempts are fruitless; it just means that you are dealing with children with children's brains. It's only when their brains mature and develop that they will be able to think and act in a way akin to an adult. Until this happens, continue to mediate when you're really needed, sit on your hands and bite your tongue as much as possible, practise the self-care tips in the previous chapter (see pages 233–234) and keep reminding yourself that sibling rivalry is normal, common and has many positives for the children.

What if they remain indifferent?

The previous chapter looked at the issue of children being indifferent towards the new baby (see page 221). Usually, this is something that wears off naturally as the baby grows into a toddler and becomes more interesting. Sometimes, however, the indifference can persist, or rather the children grow up as neither friend nor foe. This can often be as hard for parents to cope with as dealing with constantly fighting siblings. They wonder how they prevented a good sibling bond from forming – what they did wrong. And the answer is usually nothing, nothing at all.

Some siblings live very individual lives under the same roof. This tends to happen when the children don't share common interests – maybe because of a large age gap, or they are a different sex or, usually, just because they are very different children who like different things. This doesn't mean that their relationship will always be this way though. Things can, and do, change as they get older. Some siblings are as thick as thieves from the outset, but for others it can take many years before they want to spend time in each other's company. I remember my father telling me about his upbringing and how he didn't really consider his brother a friend when they were children. They didn't *not* get along, but his brother was quite a bit older than him and they just had very different lives, so it took until early adulthood for them to share common ground and really forge a strong bond. This isn't uncommon and it's not a problem that needs solving. The answer, as with so many parenting dilemmas, is patience and time. Adopting the strategies below will also help.

Five top tips to take the edge off sibling rivalry and encourage a strong sibling bond

The following tips can all help to forge a closer, more positive sibling relationship.

1. **Don't compare them.** Comparing children is possibly the most destructive thing that parents of two or more children can do. If you have a sibling, how many times did you hear your parents say things like, 'Why can't you be good, like your sister?' or, 'Your brother is so much easier than you'? How did this make you feel? Resentful? Hurt? Angry? Comparison can not only drive a wedge between parents and children, but also cause animosity between siblings. Labelling children can have similar unexpected negative consequences. Be careful not to refer to them as 'the naughty one', 'the quiet one', 'the easy one' and so on. Aside from encouraging a self-fulfilling prophecy

with the limiting beliefs that accompany labelling, the implicit comparison can often cause them to fight to keep their place or transfer the label to another member of the family. Your children are individuals – treat them as such, and the more you do, the less chance there will be of any feelings of resentment between them.

2. **Promote personal space.** Most children struggle with an invasion of their space. Toddlers on a playdate can lash out and hit a peer who tries to join them in a favourite activity, and teenagers can be hugely territorial over their belongings, albeit their lashing out is usually more verbal than physical. So helping siblings to establish their own sacred personal space is vital. As is teaching all members of the family to respect it. 'Don't touch without asking' should be a rule that applies to all. If your living arrangements don't allow for your children to have their own bedrooms, make sure that each has a special corner of a room that is theirs and theirs alone. When they are young, I recommend providing each child with their own toy box – a closed space that their sibling is not allowed to touch without their permission. As the parent, you must make sure that this is respected; don't force children to share with their siblings if they are struggling with feelings of invasion of space and a lack of ownership.

3. **Ensure you have one-to-one time.** Do you remember wondering how you would ever be able to love another child as much as your firstborn when you were expecting your second? (This is something that was covered right at the start of this book.) Then the new baby was born, and you wondered why you ever worried – maybe not immediately, but as the days and weeks went on. While love multiplies and we somehow find it in our hearts to have more than enough love for another child, our availability, sadly,

does not. American author Anthony P. Witham once said, 'Children spell love T-I-M-E'. And it couldn't be more true. While you know you love your children equally (albeit not necessarily at any given moment in time – which is totally fine by, the way), this is a worry that they struggle with throughout childhood. Making individual time for each child, one-to-one, is critical. Children need time alone with their parents, without their siblings around. This means leaving the new baby with your partner while you dash to the park with your toddler for fifteen minutes, spending a day out shopping with your teenager, while their younger sibling stays at home or taking fifteen minutes every day to tuck up each of your children in bed, in turn, rather than sharing bedtime. You may be thinking, 'But I don't have time for that!', but I think it's always possible to grab a few minutes each day. It's about utilising and prioritising time, and asking for help if you are a single parent or if your partner works away from home a lot. The sad truth is that if you don't make time for one-to-one attention for your children as they grow, then you're going to have to make time to deal with the rivalry and fights that result from not doing it. And it's much more enjoyable and easier to spend the time reconnecting with children than it is dealing with the fallout of them feeling disconnected from you and resentful of their sibling.

4. **Foster problem solving.** As discussed on page 242, your role should be that of a mediator, not a judge. Often, parents jump in and try to deal with sibling squabbles far too soon. This fix-it approach inhibits the siblings' ability to learn how to solve their own issues. Instead of jumping in and delivering a verdict, it's much better to act in a mediator-type role. See your position as encouraging communication and empathy, giving both children a

chance to feel heard, then collaboratively problem solve to reach an amicable solution. Remember, this usually means biting your tongue, while you wait for the children to work things out, with a few added pointers along the way, as in the worked example on page 242. This approach does take some practice and requires a lot of patience on your part, but it really does help, albeit probably not as quickly as you would hope.

5. **Encourage co-operative games.** Encouraging siblings to work as a team during play is a great way to transpose these skills to everyday life. Instead of encouraging games where they work against each other, racing to find a winner (and a loser), try to find ones where they work as a team towards a common goal. For younger children, co-operative board games work well (see Resources, page 270, for recommendations). For older tweens and teens, consider a family trip to an escape room, where you work together as a family to solve the clues and get out of the room. (It's expensive but you can often find special offers on ticket prices on discount deal websites.) Siblings will always disagree and fight, but with a little bit of mindful guidance, not only can you encourage their bond, but you will also help them to navigate relationship difficulties that they will come across as adults, from romantic ones to workplace ones. Remember, sibling fighting is actually a good thing for your children's emotional development.

I'd like to end this chapter with a story from a mum of two. Maddy talks about sibling rivalry developing between her two children, and how she and her partner learned to not compare or label the children and incorporate some one-to-one time, allowing each of them to feel equally special.

Maddy's story

Eight months after giving birth to my son I was pregnant again with my daughter, giving them a seventeen-month age gap. During the initial stages, my son was unfazed by his sister's presence. He would toddle over, give her a kiss and then go on his merry way. He loved making her laugh and would do silly things over and over, until he'd achieved his desired result. I was quite surprised at the way they interacted, genuinely enjoying each other's company, and thought I had 'gotten away' without any sibling jealousy.

It soon became clear, however, that rivalry was going to be a problem. My daughter had this big older brother that she wanted to keep up with and she was not going to be out-done. She reached her milestones with tenacity – crawling, walking, jumping and talking. It became clear that he felt he needed to 'up his game' but how could he achieve that when he felt Mummy and Daddy were constantly praising her efforts and ignoring his? I realised that we needed to make him feel just as important and that his achievements were just as valid. We toned down the overenthusiastic clapping and 'well dones' to our daughter while in his presence and made sure we noted the smaller things that he did. Soon, building train tracks, putting puzzles together and learning to flip on the trampoline were all met with meaningful praise and recognition. We made sure that he was not living in her shadow by getting him to show her things he could do and then saying, 'Thank you for showing her. That was really kind of you.' His smiles were worth the changes.

Soon, he enjoyed helping her achieve what he could do – but often with a little nod to how he could do it first! When the arguments came, we reminded them how lucky they were to have each other as playmates and encouraged the notion that they were best friends. Whenever they helped each other to do something I said, 'What a lovely brother/sister you are' and told them that they have beautiful hearts.

Once a month my husband and I will split off with one child each and give them quality time doing whatever they want. This allows them to be individual with their interests and means we can give the undivided attention and praise they seek. It also means that when they reunite they are excited to hear about each other's days. Now, at five years seven months and four years two months, my daughter is still lapping at his heels, but their interests are changing, and they are no longer competing for the top spot. They have a truly wonderful relationship and are happy to spend time together – often cooking up mischief!

As parents, I think most of us have a desire to fix everything in our children's worlds. We want them to be happy and well behaved, and so we struggle when we see siblings fight. The term 'sibling rivalry' is incredibly negative, setting the children up as adversaries, fighting on opposing sides. I believe we have viewed sibling fighting as problematic for too long. Rather than trying to fix squabbles and disagreements between siblings, we would be better off accepting them, understanding that they are common, normal and helpful for our children, not damaging. Taking this viewpoint is far more realistic and helps not only the children, but us too, by removing some of the stress we can so often feel when we question our children's behaviour. So the next time your children fight, take a breath, stand back and remind yourself that their disagreement is great for their future emotional health and communication skills, and feel proud that you have given them this opportunity.

Chapter 12

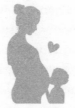

Your Feelings in the Future

I had originally planned to end this book with the previous chapter. After all, it was all about children's relationships as they grow older, and surely that's where thinking about life with two children ends? But I had doubts. Was it really the end? What does the end look like? And the more I asked myself this, the more I thought, it doesn't end. There is no ending. At least not for us as parents – or mothers, in particular. You see, it doesn't matter if your second child was born five days or fifty years ago; I think that transition always lives in you, along with the feelings that it first brought.

Certainly, almost fifteen years after my own transition from a first- to a second-time mother, I still have days when I question our decisions, and I most definitely have days when I still feel guilty. 'The Guilt' is something that needs to be talked about more, and so I decided being honest with you, with this chapter, was the best thing I could do, even if it's a tough read now.

Do you ever stop feeling guilty?

There is a quick and simple answer to this question. No. Does the guilt lessen? Absolutely! Even when my children are having a huge fight, I know, beyond any doubt, that what I did for my eldest by giving him siblings is the most precious gift I could have given him, even if he doesn't fully appreciate that yet.

I can go months, now, if not years, without feeling guilt at all. Then it hits me, out of the blue: The Guilt. It's back. It sneaks in unannounced, like an unwelcome, toxic old friend I thought I'd managed to rid myself of years ago. Just last week, I found some photo albums of my children as babies and toddlers. My firstborn's album is a beautiful blue satin. It contains hundreds of photos, neatly laid out. I have photos of his first smile, his first steps, his first Christmas, first birthday, first playgroup . . . A well-documented infancy, by a proud mum, who devoted her whole life to her baby. My second-born's album is not quite as beautiful; it was less expensive as money was tighter then. Plus, half of the pages are blank, staring at me accusingly: 'You weren't a good enough mum to fill this album up'. I have no 'firsts' in it, just snatched moments that I can't quite place. My second-born looks happy, but the album shows me quite how much of his babyhood I missed compared to that of his brother. Looking at it, I felt guilty that I didn't drink him in as much, that I didn't take as many photos, that I can't remember his firsts. I wallowed in feelings of guilt for a good half an hour, before I pulled myself together and told myself to stop being silly – that the boys never even looked at their baby albums, had no recollection of their 'firsts', or their babyhoods at all; that they couldn't care less that their photo albums are different and probably never will; that they live in the present only. It's a lesson I could learn well from them.

So I have concluded that you can never really say good-bye to the guilt – not permanently; it's more of a 'goodbye for now' than 'goodbye for ever'. As you get older, wiser and more pragmatic, the guilt lessens, the memories fade and you can talk yourself out of the feelings in ways that you never could in the early days. In a way, guilt becomes something that you live with, but accept and no longer fight or fear. I know, in my heart of hearts, that having two (and then more) children was the right thing to do, and so the benefit of experience allows me to let the grief exist, but not to feel pain or self-doubt from it any more. I'm sure there are parents who feel little guilt in the early days and none at all in the years that follow, and I think that's OK too because we're all different. The point is, however you feel – and whenever you feel it – is OK.

What about the taboo of favourite children?

Over the years, my children have often asked me who my favourite is. My answer is always the same: 'I genuinely don't have a favourite. Sometimes I might *like* one of you more, or less, but that doesn't mean my love is any different.' I think we tend to mix up 'love' and 'like'. Similarly, we confuse identifying more with one child than another with favouritism. There are certainly days when I dislike one or more of my children and we struggle to get along – or rather, I dislike their behaviour. That absolutely doesn't reflect on how much I love them though. Likewise, on a given day, one child can be a breeze, wonderfully helpful and kind and I can feel a stronger connection to them *on that particular day*. But again, that is not favouritism. I think it's more than OK to admit to yourself,

'Right now, I'm finding it much easier to parent this child than the other'. That's not favouritism. Favouritism is preferring one child to another no matter how they behave.

I also find that it is easier to relate to my children who are more like me. For instance, I am a natural introvert, I prefer quiet, solitude, thinking and theorising. One of my children is so much like me in this respect, whereas the others would all fall into the extrovert camp. I find it easier to spend time with my introverted child, simply because I understand them, and they understand me. I often see introverted parents struggle to relate to their extrovert child and vice versa. This doesn't mean that I – or they – favour this child. It doesn't affect my love for them, or the others. Again, I think we need to separate the ease of relationships and favouritism.

As children get older, I think it is vital that you discuss your relationship with them, to help them to understand that needing a break from them at some time, more than their sibling, is not a reflection of your feelings. I've found that honesty and transparency are key, no matter how hard it may be to be honest. Perhaps the hardest thing of all when thinking about favouritism with your own children is reflecting on your own upbringing, especially if you felt a sibling was favoured over you. Could it be, perhaps that what you felt at the time was favouritism actually fell into one of the categories I have discussed here? So often, parenting our children is about coming to terms with how we ourselves were raised and making peace with it. If your parents are still alive and your relationship with them is strong enough, it can be really healing to discuss with them anything you viewed as favouritism in your family and to understand what they really felt. And this, in turn, has a positive impact on the relationship you have with your own children.

That special place in your heart for your firstborn

Although my firstborn is definitely not my favourite child – because, as I've said, none of them is – I can't deny that he holds a special place in my heart. He was the child who turned me into a mother and he is the only one of my children who I have shared time alone with, in the months and years before his sibling arrived. That time alone, that taught me to be a mother, will always hold some of my fondest memories. I don't think there is anything wrong with acknowledging this specialness. Having a baby for the first time is life changing and your first-born will always be the child responsible for that. That's huge, and it's hard to think that somewhere, deep inside you, that tre-mendous life event won't be filed in a folder with 'extra special' written on it. Second-time mothers can be incredibly tough on themselves, forcing themselves to deny this specialness, but there really is no need. It doesn't indicate favouritism or a lack of bonding with your second-born. It is what it is. Don't try to fight it or question it – and especially, don't feel guilty about it.

Feeling done – or not?

Although many people 'feel done' once their second baby arrives, there are others who never feel complete. I am one of the latter. Four children on and I can't imagine what it would be like to feel done. I would have another fifty babies if I could. I can't see that yearning for 'just one more' ever leaving me. Similarly, there's that lurch I get in my ovaries when I hear a newborn cry or see a brand new 'squish' being wheeled around in a pram or carried in a sling. I've come to realise that I am one of those mad, crazy older ladies who stares at strangers' new-born babies in public. I am eternally broody and have accepted I will feel this way well into my nineties.

The feeling of 'not being done yet' is something I suspect hundreds of thousands of women live with. Does it mean you should act on it? Yes, if you actually want another baby; but no, not if you're thinking of having another because you don't feel 'done' yet. If I was to do that, I would be eternally pregnant!

I asked some mums if they felt they were done or not after the birth of their second baby. This is what they said:

I knew I was done after having two. In fact, I knew I was done before she was born. It was a mainly practical decision based on my age and not wanting to go through pregnancy again.

I never felt done ... baby number three, four and soon to be number five, who's due in a few months, were all unplanned though and conceived while on the mini pill and depo injection! But my partner earns OK, we're a little tight on space but it's manageable and we've a lot of love to give in this house, so that's made our decision each time. This time will be the last though. My partner's going to have a vasectomy!

After two I don't really feel "done", but it was easier to accept that this would be it, than if we'd only had one child.

I do feel done in a way, although I wouldn't mind a third, but I don't think I would have the energy to parent a third child. And I'm now forty-two, so possibly may have more risks in pregnancy.

I don't feel done, but I don't know how much of that is to do with the fact that I was advised not to have any more.

When my second-born arrived I felt complete almost instantly. I knew that was it for our family.

In her story, Laura talks about her feelings around having another child, which, ultimately, led to the arrival of a third baby.

Laura's story

Ten years ago, when I had my first baby, I was a different person. The shock of a difficult labour followed by a very sick baby admitted to NICU left me feeling traumatised and bereft. Every horrific procedure that she undertook made my soul die a bit more and I struggled to make that bond with her as I felt myself shut down emotionally.

Just as I started to allow myself to enjoy my bright, sparkly little girl I found out I was pregnant with my second baby. Thankfully, his birth was straightforward, but with a twenty-month gap and studying at university those early years were a blur.

In the years that followed, I threw myself into bringing up my children and studying hard. Yet I felt something was missing. Perhaps it was just female hormones making me broody, or maybe I felt cheated of the opportunity to fully enjoy my children's babyhood.

That longing didn't go away, and after eight years of head-versus-heart discussions, we decided to go for it. As I type, my beautiful third baby nestles on my knee, having spent a snuggly night curled in my arms. Bonding with her has been so straightforward and natural and – despite all the obvious practical challenges – the experience is an absolute joy. Iris has allowed my heart to heal and I feel I'm able to now enjoy every precious moment with all three of my children.

Gender disappointment

Perhaps one of the biggest taboos in our society, surrounding postnatal feelings and the desire to have another baby, is the concept of gender disappointment, or when your second baby is not the sex that you had hoped for. (Note: technically, this should be termed 'sex disappointment', since sex is biologically determined, but gender is a social construct, therefore I am using the term 'gender disappointment' as this is what is most commonly used by society.)

I think gender disappointment is unfairly labelled as self-ishness or ingratitude on the part of parents. People say, 'You have two healthy children – why would you not be happy?' But I think this highlights how little our society knows about gender disappointment. Despite the hushed tones, gender preference is very real. The book *How to Choose the Sex of Your Baby* by Landrum Shettles has sold close to 2 million copies. While, in some societies, gender preference is focused on cultural beliefs and practices, in the West, I think it is about our own upbringings, the relationships we have with our parents and the gender-stereotyped world we live in.

I had always pictured myself with a little girl. I was completely thrown, therefore, when I found out my firstborn was a boy. My childhood was very stereotypically 'girly'. As an only child, I had no experience of brothers, my toys were all dolls, my bedroom was pink and frilly and I wore classically pretty dresses. Girls were all I knew. And then suddenly, I had a boy. That was OK; I was happy to learn and soon found myself immersed in a stereotyped world totally different to the one I'd known – one full of trains, dinosaurs and astronomy. I cringe now when I look back at how biased I was when dressing my son and buying him toys. I still hoped to have a girl the next time around though. When I found out my second (and third) baby was a boy, I felt a little numb. Where was the girl I had dreamed of since childhood? In a sense, it felt like mourning. Mourning for a child I always thought I would have, but who now seemed unlikely to be a reality.

Looking back, however, I think the strongest impact on my gender disappointment was the loss of my mother. My mother died when I was twenty-one and that mother–daughter relationship was stripped away from me at a very young age. My mother was not there when I got married, bought my first house or had my first baby. Somewhere inside, I think, I harboured a hope that one day I would get to recreate what I had lost so soon with my own daughter. A daughter, to me, represented more than pretty dresses and stripy tights – it represented a chance to have a mother–daughter relationship again. I know mothers who have felt similar because they did not have a good relationship with their own mother. So when son after son was born, each arrival, although joyous, involved a little bit of mourning too. I was overjoyed to have another healthy baby boy and the desire to have a girl did not impact on my love for my new son in any way, but there was always a longing, a hope, a desire and a spot of sadness that didn't leave.

When my daughter was born – my fourth baby – I expected to feel some sort of completeness. And it shocked me when I didn't. I quickly realised that the daughter that I had imagined for all those years wasn't real. The daughter I had was. She hated dresses, stripped off any tights I put her in, she never played with dolls, she gets bored after ten minutes of shopping and we have a completely different relationship to the one I had with my mother. I began to understand that, for me, it wasn't about the baby's sex at all, but about thoughts and feelings from my childhood. No child, boy or girl, was going to change that.

Does that mean I think gender disappointment is wrong?

No, absolutely not. I think it's a very real feeling that we should be more aware and supportive of, and it's sad that so little research exists on it. I don't think it's wrong to want a child of a different sex or to feel sad when the one that is born is the opposite. I do, however, think it's important to examine what is underpinning our feelings because, often, they aren't about the sex of our children at all.

Below, Jodie shares her story of gender hopes. I think the point to note here is about loving another child, no matter if they are a boy or a girl. If you find yourself wishing for a number three because you have two girls or two boys, the two most important questions you can ask yourself are: 'Do I want another child, or just a boy or a girl?' and 'What happens if it's a third boy or a third girl? Will I be as happy and love them as much?'

Jodie's story

We've always only wanted two children, as it just seemed like the perfect family number. For both pregnancies, which were two-and-a-half years apart, we didn't ask to know what the gender was and preferred a surprise at birth. In fact, not knowing the gender was a big statement for us that it didn't matter, boy or girl, as long as they were healthy.

Turns out that after the second girl was born, I didn't quite feel like our family was complete, after all. Following two years of broodiness and longing for another baby, it appears that there are some aspects of gender disappointment in that feeling. As much as it felt right at the time not caring about the gender, and as much as I love having two girls (I'm one of five and think it's amazing to have sisters), I find myself day dreaming of having a little boy as an addition to our family.

I've always heard of people who regretted not having another child, but never heard of anyone who regretted conceiving again. So now I need to exercise some convincing with my husband to try for a third child! And if all works out, and yet another girl comes – which would be equally lovely – I wonder if I'll still feel broody or if our family will finally feel complete.

Accepting that you are done at two

Whether you feel done or have decided that stopping at two children is right for your family, the decision can still bring a tinge of sadness. Stopping at two means saying goodbye to something that has been such a large part of you for so long: pregnancy, birth and early motherhood. Stopping at two children means facing your own ageing and losing a part of your identity (as a mother to young children). For some, that can be a joyous thing indeed – the realisation that they will never again have to deal with morning sickness, labour pains or sleepless nights; for others, it's a bittersweet resolution.

I think the best way to move forwards, if the thought brings you more sadness than joy, is to work on reclaiming yourself a little. Think about who you were and what you enjoyed before having children. Consider anything that you would like to achieve in the future, whether that's learning a new hobby or retraining for a new career. And this brings us back to the discussion of self-care in Chapter 10 – nurturing yourself, in body and in mind, so that you can feel complete, fulfilled and peaceful with your family.

*

If you have read this chapter while still pregnant, or holding a newborn, I hope I haven't scared you too much. There is every likelihood that you won't feel any of the things that I have written about in it, but, on the off-chance that you do, I hope that my words will reassure you and help you to feel normal.

If you have read this chapter a little further down the line, I hope it has helped you to feel less alone and a little more sane.

A Closing Note

Each child is an adventure into a better life,
an opportunity to change the old pattern and
make it new.
    Hubert H. Humphrey Jr, American politician

I think these words are the perfect way to end this book. They describe exactly the potential and joy that a second baby can bring to a family, while also being mindful of the work needed to get ready for the transition and make it as positive as possible for all family members, even years later.

Having a second baby is hard work. It involves lots of planning and preparation, patience and compassion, both before and after the arrival. In many ways, it is a much harder transition than having a baby for the first time. The guilt, coping with your firstborn's behaviour when they struggle to adapt and the adjustments you yourself must make, can sometimes feel impossible. You have done this before though, and while you may not have experience of having two, you are also not the same green newbie that you were the first time around. This experience, combined with the advice in this book, I hope will help you to feel calmer and more excited about what is about to happen, or has happened already, in your life.

Second babies bring with them opportunity, promises of the future and a chance to create something magical – a lasting friendship for your firstborn. The first time your children truly interact, when your firstborn tenderly kisses their new baby sibling, when the baby gives their first gummy smile to their big brother or sister, rather than you and the first time they really play together, makes everything else worthwhile. Treasure these glimmers of the future friendship your children will have. Lock them in a memory box in your mind, so that you can revel in them on the days when it all feels so hard. Because, ultimately, this is what having a second baby is all about: the greatest gift you could ever give your children.

Good luck!

Sarah

Reasons-to-wait list

As discussed in Chapter 1, page 25, when weighing up the decision when – or indeed if – to have another child you may find it useful to fill in the following chart.

Reasons to wait	Importance out of 10 (10 being the most important)	Possible solutions

Reasons to wait	Importance out of 10 (10 being the most important)	Possible solutions

Resources

Sarah Ockwell-Smith

Sarah's website: www.sarahockwell-smith.com
Facebook: www.facebook.com/sarahockwellsmithauthor
Twitter: www.twitter.com/thebabyexpert
Instagram: www.instagram.com/sarahockwellsmith

Chapter Two

Weschler, Toni., *Taking Charge of Your Fertility: The Definitive Guide to Natural Birth Control, Pregnancy Achievement and Reproductive Health*, Vermilion, Revised Edition, 2016.

Human Fertilisation and Embryology Association (HFEA): www.hfea.gov.uk

Fertility UK (national fertility awareness network): www.fertilityuk.org

Fertility Network (fertility support charity): www.fertilitynetworkuk.org

Fertility Friend ovulation calendar: www.fertilityfriend.com

MIND (mental health charity): www.mind.org.uk

PANDAS Foundation (support with pre- and post-natal mental illness): www.pandasfoundation.org.uk

Chapter Three

The Lullaby Trust (emotional support for bereaved families): www.lullabytrust.org.uk

Sands (stillbirth and neonatal death charity): www.sands.org.uk

Tommy's (advice on coping with grief after the loss of a baby): www.tommys.org

JOEL (supporting families through pregnancy and parenting after the loss of a baby): www.joeltcp.org

Flower, H. and O'Mara, P., *Adventures in Tandem Nursing: Breastfeeding During Pregnancy and Beyond*, La Leche League International, 2003.

Kellymom (information on breastfeeding during pregnancy and tandem nursing): kellymom.com/ages/tandem/official-tandem-bf-faq

Chapter Four

Civardi, A. and Cartwright, S., *The New Baby*, Usborne First Experiences, Usborne, 2005.

Tapper, L. and Wilson, S., *You're the Biggest: Keepsake Gift Book Celebrating Becoming a Big Brother or Sister*, Me to You Publishing, 2017.

Overend, J. and Vivas, J., *Hello Baby*, Frances Lincoln Children's Books, 2009.

Andraea, G. and Cabban, V., *There's A House Inside my Mummy*, Orchard Books, UK edition, 2002.

Maclean, A. and Nesbitt, J., *Our Water Baby*, The Good Birth Company, 2006.

Sears, W., Sears, M. and Kelly, C., *What Baby Needs*, Little, Brown for Young Readers, 2001.

Chapter Five

Babywearing UK (social enterprise promoting the use of slings and carriers): www.babywearing.co.uk

School of Babywearing (help with finding a babywearing consultant): www.schoolofbabywearing.com/find-a-babywearing-consultant/

Trading standards product recall information: www.trading-standards.uk/consumers/product-recalls

Mexican rebozo techniques: www.spinningbabies.com/learn-more/techniques/the-fantastic-four/rebozo-manteada-sifting

Chapter Six

Birth Trauma Association: www.birthtraumaassociation.org.uk

The Positive Birth Movement: www.positivebirthmovement.org

The Hypnobirthing Association: www.thehypnobirthingassociation.com

Wise Hippo Hypnobirthing: www.thewisehippo.com

Doula UK: www.doula.org.uk

Doula access fund (information on financial help when hiring a doula): www.doula.org.uk/doula-access-fund

VBAC information: www.vbac.com

Homebirth reference site: www.homebirth.org.uk

Chapter Eight

The International Association of Infant Massage: www.iaim.org.uk

Chapter Nine

Gentle Sleep Music for Babies recording, by Ian Ockwell-Smith. Available as an MP3 download from Amazon, iTunes and Google Play.

Gentle Sleep Relaxation for Children recording, by Sarah Ockwell-Smith. Available as an MP3 download from Amazon, iTunes and Google Play.

Safe co-sleeping (bedsharing) guidelines: www.cosleeping. nd.edu/safe-co-sleeping-guidelines/

Chapter Eleven

Peaceable Kingdom co-operative games: www.mindware.com/ peaceablekingdom

Escape room directory: www.playexitgames.com

References

Chapter 1

1. Zajonc, R. B. and Markus, G. B., 'Birth order and intellectual development', *Psychological Review*, 82(1) (1975), pp. 74–88.
2. Werner, E., 'Vulnerability and resiliency: a longitudinal study of Asian Americans from birth to age 30', paper presented at the Biennial Meeting of the International Society for the Study of Behavioural Development, Tokyo, July 1987.
3. Kidwell, J., 'Number of siblings, sibling spacing, sex, and birth order: their effects on perceived parent-adolescent relationships', *Journal of Marriage and Family*, 43(2) (1981), pp. 315–32.
4. Galdikas, B. and Wood, J., 'Birth spacing patterns in humans and apes', *American Journal of Physical Anthropology*, 83(2) (1990), pp. 185–91.
5. Pennington, R., 'Hunter-gatherer demography,' in C. Panter-Brick, R. H. Layton and P. Rowley-Conwy (eds) *Hunter-Gatherers: An Interdisciplinary Perspective*, Cambridge University Press (2001), pp. 170–204.
6. Conde-Agudelo, A., Rosas-Bermudez, A. and Kafury-Goeta, A., 'Birth spacing and risk of adverse perinatal outcomes: a meta-analysis,' *Journal of the American Medical Association* 295(15) (2006), pp. 1809–23.
7. Rutstein, A., 'Further evidence of the effects of preceding birth intervals on neonatal, infant, and under-five-years mortality and nutritional status in developing countries: Evidence from the demographic health surveys', DHS Working Paper no. 41, Washington, D.C.: United States Agency for International Development (2008).
8. Ibid.

9. Getahun, D., Strickland, D. and Ananth, C., 'Recurrence of preterm premature rupture of membranes in relation to interval between pregnancies', *American Journal of Obstetrics and Gynecology*, 202(6) (2010), pp. 1–570; Bujold, E. and Gauthier, R., 'Risk of uterine rupture associated with an interdelivery interval between 18 and 24 months', *Obstetrics and Gynecology*, 115(5) (2010), pp. 1003–6; Conde-Agudelo, A., Rosas-Bermudez, A., Kafury-Goeta, A., 'Birth spacing and risk of adverse perinatal outcomes: a meta-analysis,' *Journal of the American Medical Association*, 295(15) (2006), pp. 1809–23.

10. Grundy, E. and Kravdal, O., 'Do short birth intervals have long-term implications for parental health? Results from analyses of complete cohort Norwegian register data', *Journal of Epidemiology Community Health*, 68(10) (2014), pp. 958–64.

Chapter 2

1. Steiner, A. and Jukic, A., 'Impact of female age and nulligravidity on fecundity in an older reproductive age cohort', *Fertility and Sterility*, 105 (6) (2016), pp. 1584–8.

2. Perez, A., 'Natural Family Planning: Postpartum Period', *International Journal of Fertility*, 26(3) (1981), pp. 219–21.

3. Crawford, N., Pritchard, D., Herring, A. and Steiner, A., 'Prospective evaluation of luteal phase length and natural fertility', *Fertility and Sterility*, 107(3) (2017), pp. 749–55.

4. Howie, P., 'Natural regulation of fertility', *British Medical Bulletin*, 49(1) (1993), pp. 182–99.

5. Heinig, M., Nommsen-Rivers, L., Peerson, J. and Dewey, K., 'Factors related to duration of postpartum amenorrhoea among USA women with prolonged lactation', *Journal of Biosocial Science*, 26(4) (1994), pp. 517–27.

6. Perez, A., 'Natural Family Planning: Postpartum Period', *International Journal of Fertility*, 26(3) (1981), pp. 219–21.

7. Heinig, M., Nommsen-Rivers, L., Peerson, J. and Dewey, K., 'Factors related to duration of postpartum amenorrhoea among USA women with prolonged lactation', *Journal of Biosocial Science*, 26(4) (1994), pp. 517–27.

8. McNeilly, A., Glasier, A., Howie, P., Houston, M., Cook, A. and Boyle, H., 'Fertility after childbirth: pregnancy associated with breast feeding', *Clinical Endocrinology*, 19(2) (1983), pp. 167–73.

9. Best, D., Avenell, A. and Bhattacharya, S., 'How effective are weight-loss interventions for improving fertility in women and

men who are overweight or obese? A systematic review and meta-analysis of the evidence', *Human Reproduction Update*, 23(6) (2017), pp. 681–705.

10. Grieger, J., et al., https://www.ncbi.nlm.nih.gov/pubmed/2973 3398 'Pre-pregnancy fast food and fruit intake is associated with time to pregnancy', *Human Reproduction*, 33(6) (2018), pp. 1063–70.

11. Hayden, R., Flannigan, R. and Schelgel, R., https://www.ncbi. nlm.nih.gov/pubmed/29774489 'The role of lifestyle in male infertility: diet, physical activity, and body habitus', *Current Urology Reports*, 19(7) (2018), p. 56; Sharma, R., Biedenharn, K. and Agarwal, A., 'Lifestyle factors and reproductive health: taking control of your fertility', *Reproductive Biology and Endocrinology*, 11(66) (2013).

12. Durairaianayagam, D., 'Lifestyle causes of male infertility', *Arab Journal of Urology*, 16(1) (2018), pp. 10–20.

13. Camlin, N., McLaughlin, E. and Holt, J., 'Through the smoke: use of in vivo and in vitro cigarette smoking models to elucidate its effect on female fertility', *Toxicology and Applied Pharmacology*, 281(3) (2014), pp. 266–75.

14. Wang, I., et al., 'Non-apnea sleep disorder increases the risk of subsequent female infertility – a nationwide population-based cohort study', *Sleep*, 41(1) (2018).

15. Wise, L., Rothman, K., Wesselink, A., Mikkelsen, E., Sorensen, H., McKinnon, C. and Hatch, E., 'Male sleep duration and fecundability in a North American preconception cohort study', *Fertility and Sterility*, 109(3): (2018), pp. 453–9.

16. Robinson, J. and Ellis, J., 'Mistiming of intercourse as a primary cause of failure to conceive: results of a survey on use of a home-use fertility monitor', *Current Medical Research and Opinion*, 23 (2007), pp. 301–6.

17. Robinson, J., Wakelin, M. and Ellis J., 'Increased pregnancy rate with the use of the Clearblue Easy fertility monitor', *Fertility and Sterility*, 87(2) (2007), pp. 329–34.

18. Wilcox, A., Weinber, C. and Baird, D., 'Timing of sexual intercourse in relation to ovulation: effects on the probability of conception, survival of the pregnancy, and sex of the baby', *New England Journal of Medicine*, 333(23) (1996), pp.1517–21.

19. Frank-Herrmann, P., Jacobs, C., Jenetzky, E., et al., 'Natural conception rates in subfertile couples following fertility awareness training', *Archives of Gyneacology and Obstetrics*, 295(4) (April 2017), pp. 1015–24.

20. Bushnik, T., Cook, J., Yuzpe, A., Tough, S. and Collins, J., 'Estimating the prevalence of infertility in Canada', *Human Reproduction*, 27(3) (2012), pp. 738–46.

Chapter 3

1. Biaggi, A., Conroy, S., Pawlby, A. and Pariante, C., 'Identifying the women at risk of antenatal anxiety and depression: a systematic review', *Journal of Affective Disorders*, 191 (2016), pp. 62–77.
2. Ibid.
3. Wilcox, M., Chang, A. and Johnson, I., 'The effects of parity on birthweight using successive pregnancies', *Acta Obstetricia et Gynecologica Scandinavica*, 75(5) (1996), pp. 459–63.
4. Mittendorf, R., Williams, M., Berkey, C. and Cotter, P., 'The length of uncomplicated human gestation', *Obstetrics and Gynecology*, 75(6) (1990), pp. 929–32.

Chapter 4

1. Wright, H. and Lack, L., 'Effect of light wavelength on suppression and phase delay of the melatonin rhythm', *Chronobiology International*, 18(5) (2001), pp. 801–8.
2. Akacem, L., Wright, K. and LeBourgeois, M., 'Sensitivity of the circadian system to evening bright light in preschool-age children', *Physiological Reports*, 6(5) (2018).
3. Nakagawa, M., et al., 'Daytime nap controls toddlers' nighttime sleep', *Scientific Reports*, 6, article no. 27246 (2016).
4. LeBourgeois, M., Wright, K., LeBourgeois, H. and Jenni, O., 'Dissonance between parent-selected bedtimes and young children's circadian physiology influences nighttime settling difficulties', *Mind Brain and Education*, 7(4) (2013), pp. 234–42.
5. Gunnar, M., Larson, M., Hertsgaard, L., Harris, M. and Brodersen, L., 'The stressfulness of separation among 9-month-old infants: effects of social context variables and infant temperament', *Child Development*, 63 (1992), pp. 290–303.
6. Ishii, H., 'Does breastfeeding induce spontaneous abortion?', *Journal of Obstetrics and Gynaecology Research*, 35(5) (2009), pp. 864–8.
7. Madarshahian, F., Hassanibadi, M., 'A comparative study of breastfeeding during pregnancy: impact on maternal and newborn outcomes', *Journal of Nursing Research*, 20(1) (2012), pp. 74–80.

Chapter 5

1. Tappin, D., Brooke, H., Ecob, R. and Gibson, A., 'Used infant mattresses and sudden infant death syndrome in Scotland: case-control study', *British Medical Journal*, 325(7371) (2002), p. 1007.

Chapter 6

1. Elvander, C., Dahlberg, J., Andersson, G. and Cnattingius, S., 'Mode of delivery and the probability of subsequent childbearing: a population-based register study', *International Journal of Obstetrics and Gynecology*,122(12) (2015), pp. 1593–1600.
2. Anim-Somuah, M., Smyth, R. and Howell, C., 'Epidural versus non-epidural or no analgesia in labour', *Cochrane Database of Systematic Reviews*, (4) (2005).
3. Yogev, Y., Hiersch, L., Maresky, L., Wasserberg, N. and Melamed, N., 'Third and fourth degree perineal tears – the risk of recurrence in subsequent pregnancy', *Journal of Maternal and Fetal Neonatal Medicine*, 27(2) (2014), pp. 177–81.
4. Lee, T., Carpenter, M., Heber, W. and Silver, H., 'Preterm premature rupture of membranes: risks of recurrent complications in the next pregnancy among a population-based sample of gravid women', *American Journal of Obstetrics and Gynecology*, 188(1) (2003), pp. 209–13.
5. Ghomian, N., Hafizi, L. and Takhti, Z., 'The role of vitamin C in prevention of preterm premature rupture of membranes', *Iranian Red Crescent Medical Journal*, 15(2) (2013), pp. 113–16.
6. Mittendorf, R., Williams, M., Berkey, C. and Cotter, P., 'The length of uncomplicated human gestation', *Obstetrics and Gynecology*, 75(6) (1990), pp. 929–32.
7. Office for National Statistics, 'Birth characteristics in England and Wales', Statistical Bulletin (2015).
8. Janssen, P., Saxell, L., Page, L., Klein, M., Liston, R. and Lee, S., 'Outcomes of planned home birth with registered midwife versus planned hospital birth with midwife or physician', *Canadian Medical Association Journal*, 181(6-7) (2009), pp. 377–83.
9. Landon, M. B., Spong, C. Y., Thom, E., Hauth, J. C., Bloom, S. L., Varner, M. W., et al., 'Risk of uterine rupture with a trial of labor in women with multiple and single prior cesarean delivery', *Obstetrics and Gynecology*, 108 (2006), pp. 12–20.
10. Dekker, G. A., Chan, A., Luke, C. G., Priest, K., Riley, M.,

Halliday, J., et al., 'Risk of uterine rupture in Australian women attempting vaginal birth after one prior caesarean section: a retrospective population-based cohort study', *British Journal of Obstetrics and Gynaecology*,117 (2010), pp. 1358–65.

11.   https://www.rcog.org.uk/globalassets/documents/guidelines/ gtg_45.pdf

12.   Guise, J. M., Eden, K., Emeis, C., Denman, M. A., Marshall, N., Fu, R., et al., 'Vaginal birth after cesarean: new insights. Evidence reports/technology assessments', no. 191, Rockville, Maryland, USA: Agency for Healthcare Research and Quality (2010).

13.   Jozwiak, M. and Dodd, J. M., 'Methods of term labour induction for women with a previous caesarean section', *Cochrane Database of Systematic Reviews*, (3) (2013).

14.   Devane, D., Lalor, J. G., Daly, S., McGuire, W., Cuthbert, A. and Smith, V., 'Comparing electronic monitoring of the baby's heartbeat on a woman's admission in labour using cardiotocography (CTG) with intermittent monitoring', *Cochrane Database of Systematic Reviews*, (2017).

15.   Rowe, R., Li, Y.,Knight, M., Brocklehurst, P., Hollowell, J., 'Maternal and perinatal outcomes in women planning vaginal birth after caesarean (VBAC) at home in England: secondary analysis of the Birthplace national prospective cohort study', *British Journal of Obstetrics and Gynaecology*, 123(7) (2015), pp. 1123-32.

16.   Nutter, E., Meyer, S., Shaw-Battista, J. and Marowitz, A., 'Waterbirth: an integrative analysis of peer-reviewed literature', *Journal or Midwifery and Women's Health*, 59(3) (2014), pp. 286–319.

17.   Smith, J., Plaat, F. and Fisk, N., 'The natural caesarean: a woman-centred technique', *British Journal of Obstetrics and Gynaecology*, 115(8) (2008): pp. 1037–1042.

18.   Plain Language Summaries, 'Pain relief for after pains (uterine cramping/involution) after the baby's birth' *Cochrane Database of Systematic Reviews* (2011).

Chapter 11

1.   http://toddlersup.wixsite.com/toddlersup.

Index

(page numbers in *italics* relate to illustrations)